Synthesis Lectures on Technology and Health

The series publishes state-of-the-art short books on transformative technologies for health, wellness, and independent living. Our scope of publishing in the expanding health tech field includes:

- Technology in support of active and healthy living and aging
- Digital technologies for health- and social-care improvement
- Diagnostic, screening, and tracking tools
- Assistive and rehabilitative technologies

The series includes a subseries of books published in partnership with Canada's AGE-WELL that specifically addresses their 8 AgeTech Challenge Areas. Each lecture introduces the context in which the technology is used—wellness, health, medicine, special needs, or other contexts. Authors present and explain the technology and review promising applications and opportunities as well as limitations and challenges. They include material on their own work while surveying the broader landscape of related research, development, and impact.

Amara Callistus Nwosu · Sarah Stanley ·
James Norris · Mark Taubert

Technologies in Palliative Care for Older People

AGEWELL

Springer

Amara Callistus Nwosu
Lancaster Medical School
Lancaster University
Lancaster, UK

James Norris
MyWishes
Michael Sobell House, Mount Vernon Hospital
Northwood, London, UK

Sarah Stanley
Liverpool John Moores University
Liverpool, UK

Mark Taubert
Palliative Care Department
Velindre Cancer Centre
Cardiff, UK

ISSN 2771-7054 ISSN 2771-7070 (electronic)
Synthesis Lectures on Technology and Health
ISBN 978-3-032-04276-7 ISBN 978-3-032-04277-4 (eBook)
https://doi.org/10.1007/978-3-032-04277-4

This Springer imprint is published by the registered company Springer Nature Switzerland AG
The registered company address is: Gewerbestrasse 11, 6330 Cham, Switzerland

Acknowledgements

The authors would like to thank the Science and Technology for Aging Research (STAR) Institute, of Simon Fraser University, for its administrative and financial support, and AGE-WELL for its financial support.

The authors would particularly like to thank the AGE-WELL community—The Network Management Office, researchers, older adults and caregivers, and partners. Their passion for innovation was essential in developing and sustaining this book's creation. Thank you for your collaborative spirit.

The authors express their appreciation to Andrew Sixsmith and Juliet Neun-Hornick for their excellent support in the development of the book. The authors offer their gratitude to the Springer publishing team for their deep knowledge and professionalism.

Dr. Amara Nwosu would like to thank his colleagues at Lancaster University, Marie Curie Hospice Liverpool, Liverpool University Hospitals NHS Foundation Trust and the Churchill Fellowship, who have supported him during the writing of this book. Amara thanks his parents (Cally and Beverley) for their unwavering love and support.

Sarah Stanley would like to thank the inspirational patients, caregivers and bereaved caregivers who have contributed invaluably to her digital health research, and have shown the importance of carrying out research in this area.

James Norris would like to thank colleagues at the Digital Legacy Association and MyWishes. A special thank you and acknowledgement is provided to Dr. Ros Taylor MBE for her ongoing, altruistic support and guidance.

Professor Mark Taubert would like to thank and remember Dr. Kate Granger MBE, who got him into the world of health-related technology and social media in the first place.

All the authors would like to dedicate this book to all patients, families and caregivers who are affected by serious illness. Our hope is that the content of this book can support the science and art of delivering patient-focused care and to determine how society can best use technology to improve palliative care for older people.

Certain photographs used in this publication are from The Centre for Aging Better, Age-Positive Image Library. For further details, visit: https://agingbetter.resourcespace.com/pages/search.php.

AGE-WELL (www.agewell-nce.ca) is Canada's Technology and Aging Network. The pan-Canadian network brings together researchers, older adults, caregivers, partner organizations, and future leaders to accelerate the delivery of technology-based solutions that make a meaningful difference in the lives of Canadians. AGE-WELL researchers are producing technologies, services, policies, and practices that improve quality of life for older adults and caregivers, and generate social and economic benefits for Canada. AGE-WELL's work is supported through Government of Canada funding programs.

The STAR (Science and Technology for Aging Research) Institute (www.sfu.ca/starinstitute) at Simon Fraser University (SFU) is committed to supporting community-engaged research in the rapidly growing area of technology and aging. The Institute supports the development and implementation of technologies to address many of the health challenges encountered in old age, as well as addresses the social, commercial, and policy aspects of using and accessing technologies. STAR also supports the AGE-WELL network.

AGEWELL

STAR INSTITUTE
Science and Technology for Aging Research
Simon Fraser University

Contents

About the Authors

Dr. Amara Callistus Nwosu is a Senior Clinical Lecturer in Palliative Care at Lancaster University, and Research Lead for Marie Curie North West. Amara is an Honorary Clinical Consultant in Palliative Care at Liverpool University Hospitals NHS Foundation Trust. Amara is an Honorary Senior Clinical Lecturer at the University of Liverpool. Amara's research focuses on digital health in palliative care. In 2023, Amara completed a Churchill Fellowship in the USA and the Netherlands, researching palliative care digital health.

Sarah Stanley is a research nurse at Marie Curie UK. Sarah is experienced in palliative care nursing and clinical research. In 2018, Sarah received the Marie Curie Susie Wilkinson Award in recognition of her research development. Sarah is undertaking a Ph.D. at Liverpool John Moores University, which explores digital legacy in end-of-life care advance care planning from the perspective of service users, caregivers, bereaved people and healthcare professionals.

James Norris is an 'End of Life Technologist' and founded the not-for-profit, Digital Legacy Association (DLA) in 2015. James conducts research, training, and develops areas of best practice in digital assets planning and digital legacy safeguarding at the DLA. James is the founder of MyWishes, a public health intervention, that provides digital approaches to advance care planning and end of life planning. James is based at Harlington Hospice's Inpatient Unit, Michael Sobell House, in North London.

Prof. Mark Taubert is a hospital consultant and clinical director at Velindre Cancer Service in Cardiff, Wales. He has academic roles at Cardiff University, is the founder of TalkCPR.com, and chairs the national Future Care Planning strategy group for the National Health Service in Wales. Mark is the Vice-President of the European Association for Palliative Care, a Brussels-based Non-Governmental Organization (NGO). Mark is a fellow of the Learned Society of Wales.

Abbreviations and Acronyms

ACP	Advance Care Planning
AI	Artificial Intelligence
AR	Augmented Reality
BBC	British Broadcasting Corporation
CAPC	Center to Advance Palliative Care
CMC	Coordinate my Care
COPD	Chronic Obstructive Pulmonary Disease
CPR	Cardio Pulmonary Resuscitation
CT	Computed Tomography
DNACPR	Do not Attempt Cardiopulmonary Resuscitation
ECHO	Extension of Community Healthcare Outcomes
EIP	European Innovation Partnership
EPR	Electronic Patient Records
EU	European Union
GP	General Practitioner
ICT	Information and Communication Technologies
IoT	Internet of Things
IMPaCT	Integrated Mersey Palliative Care Team
IT	Information Technology
ML	Machine Learning
MR	Mixed Reality
MRI	Magnetic Resonance Imaging
NIHR	National Institute for Health and Care Research
NHS	National Health Service
NLP	Natural Language Processing
RPA	Robotic Process Automation
RPM	Remote Patient Monitoring
SCS	Spinal Cord Stimulation

SICP	Serious Illness Care Program
SMS	Short Message Service
TENS	Transcutaneous Electrical Nerve Stimulation
VR	Virtual Reality
UK	United Kingdom
WHO	World Health Organizatiion

1 Introduction and Overview to the Book

1.1 The Challenge

AgeTech refers to the use of advanced technologies such as information and communication technologies (ICTs), robotics, mobile technologies, artificial intelligence (AI), ambient systems and pervasive computing, to drive technology-based innovation to benefit older adults (Pruchno, 2019). Cross-disciplinary research demonstrates the potential of AgeTech to transform the delivery of health and social care and improve patient-centred outcomes (Topol, 2019; Department of Health Social Care, 2018; Haghi et al., 2017). AgeTech is increasingly important in enabling older adults to manage their health and well-being (Sixsmith et al., 2017). Furthermore, healthcare providers are increasingly using AgeTech to support communication, diagnosis, prevention and treatments of health issues affecting older citizens (Nkhoma et al., 2021) (Fig. 1.1).

Palliative care describes a model of care that improves the quality-of-life of patients and their families facing the problems associated with life-threatening illness (World Health Organization, 2010). Global palliative care need is increasing due to several socioeconomic factors, such as population aging (Sleeman et al., 2019). There is limited data describing how AgeTech can be meaningfully used, by service users and healthcare professionals, to support the palliative care needs of older people. Furthermore, there is a lack understanding of how healthcare organizations and systems should use AgeTech (from a design and coordination perspective), to ensure the needs of patients are adequately addressed as they evolve throughout illness, as their physical health deteriorates (Murray et al., 2005).

AgeTech has unmet potential in supporting the palliative care needs of older people. This is because most AgeTech applications are designed to support older people to maintain physical function, prevent ill-health and promote independence, rather than respond to the evolving care needs of worsening health (Bertolazzi et al., 2024). Consequently,

A. C. Nwosu et al., *Technologies in Palliative Care for Older People*, Synthesis Lectures on Technology and Health, https://doi.org/10.1007/978-3-032-04277-4_1

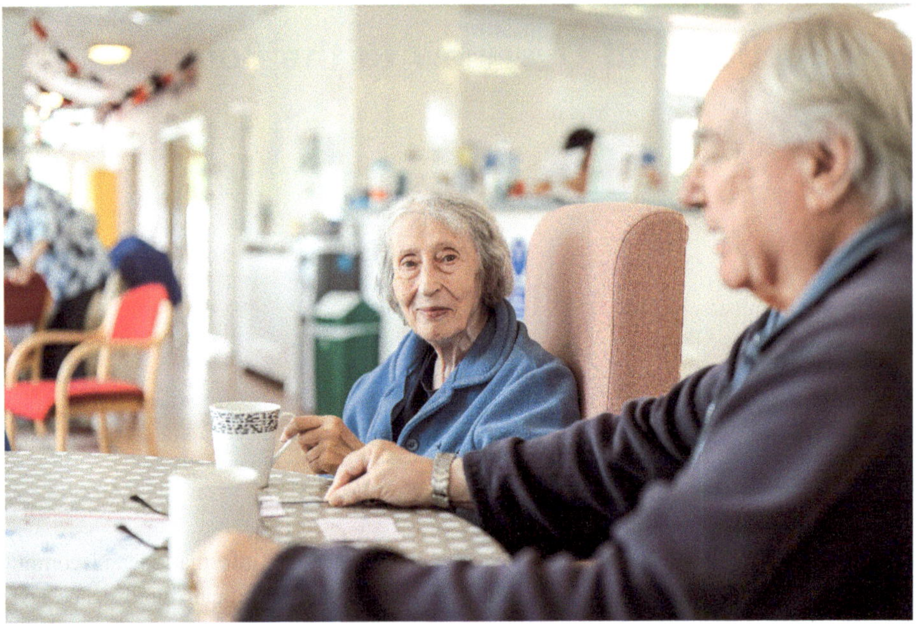

Fig. 1.1 *Credit* Bramley elderly action/aging better

some AgeTech technologies cease to be helpful for older people who develop increasing physical and psychosocial care needs, especially if the AgeTech tools no longer meet the requirements of the user (e.g., someone with cancer may lose the ability to operate their tablet due to decreased hand dexterity caused by fatigue) (Nwosu, 2023). Therefore, it is important to examine the opportunities and challenges of using AgeTech for older people who experience increasing palliative care need as they age (Nwosu, 2023). To address this issue, this book explores the potential to use AgeTech to support the palliative care needs of older people, according to their specific needs. We highlight the opportunities and challenges associated with relevant technologies, and we consider the human-related factors, which are important to evaluate how AgeTech can support the evolving needs of older people.

1.2 Overview of the Book

The aim of this book is to provide health practitioners, academics, and students (who are interested in technology and aging) with an accessible overview of developments of how AgeTech technologies can potentially support the delivery of palliative care for older people (Fig. 1.2).

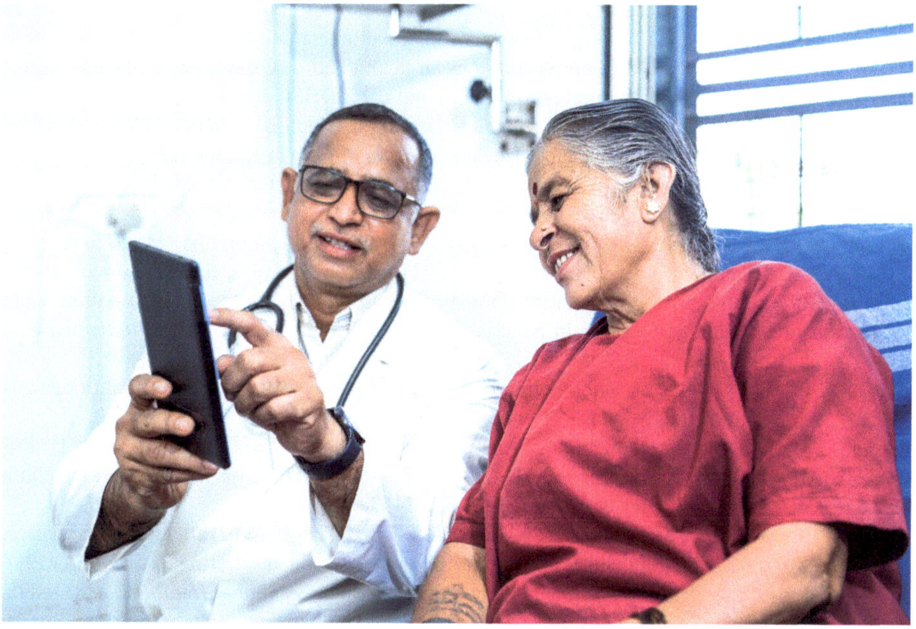

Fig. 1.2 *Credit* Westock productions/Shutterstock

This book is written to be accessible for readers from a several disciplines, focusing on describing issues related to aging and palliative care. We begin with an overview of the origins of palliative care, by describing the hospice movement, and its significance to older people and aging. We then describe developments in AgeTech, highlighting its potential to support palliative care needs of older people, and the associated opportunities and challenges. In the following chapters, we present a user-centred perspective of how AgeTech can potentially address the specific problems associated with aging and palliative care. We conclude this book by describing the future scenarios and implications (practical, research and policy) for stakeholders to consider when identifying how AgeTech can support the palliative care needs of older people.

References

Bertolazzi, A., Quaglia, V. & Bongelli, R. 2024. Barriers and facilitators to health technology adoption by older adults with chronic diseases: an integrative systematic review. *BMC public health*, 24, 506.

Clark, D. 2007. From margins to centre: a review of the history of palliative care in cancer. *Lancet Oncol*, 8, 430–438.

Department of health social care 2018. The future of healthcare: our vision for digital, data and technology in health and care. https://www.gov.uk/government/publications/the-future-of-healthcare-our-vision-for-digital-data-and-technology-in-health-and-care/the-future-of-healthcare-our-vision-for-digital-data-and-technology-in-health-and-care: DHSC London.

Haghi, M., Thurow, K. & Stoll, R. 2017. Wearable Devices in Medical Internet of Things: Scientific Research and Commercially Available Devices. *Healthc Inform Res*, 23, 4–15.

Murray, S. A., Kendall, M., Boyd, K. & Sheikh, A. 2005. Illness trajectories and palliative care. *BMJ*, 330, 1007–1011.

Nkhoma, K. B., Ebenso, B., Akeju, D., Adejoh, S., Bennett, M., Chirenje, M., Dandadzi, A., Nabirye, E., Namukwaya, E. & Namisango, E. 2021. Stakeholder perspectives and requirements to guide the development of digital technology for palliative cancer services: a multi-country, cross-sectional, qualitative study in Nigeria, Uganda and Zimbabwe. *BMC palliative care*, 20, 1–16.

Nwosu, A. C. 2023. Telehealth requires improved evidence to achieve its full potential in palliative care. SAGE Publications Sage UK: London, England.

Pruchno, R. 2019. Technology and aging: An evolving partnership. *The Gerontologist*, 59(1), 1–5.

Sixsmith, A., Mihailidis, A. & Simeonov, D. 2017. Aging and technology: Taking the research into the real world. *Public Policy & Aging Report*, 27, 74–78.

Sleeman, K. E., De Brito, M., Etkind, S., Nkhoma, K., Guo, P., Higginson, I. J., Gomes, B. & Harding, R. 2019. The escalating global burden of serious health-related suffering: projections to 2060 by world regions, age groups, and health conditions. *The Lancet Global Health*, 7, e883–e892.

Topol, E. 2019. Preparing the Healthcare Workforce to Deliver the Digital Future the Topol Review: An Independent Report on Behalf of the Secretary of State for Health and Social Care. *NHS Health Education: London, UK*.

World Health Organization 1990. Cancer pain relief and palliative care. *WHO Technical Report Series 804*.

World Health Organization. 2010. *WHO Definition of Palliative Care* [Online]. Available: http://www.who.int/cancer/palliative/definition/en/ [Accessed].

2 Palliative Care and Older People

2.1 What is Palliative Care?

Palliative care is important to provide holistic, person-centered support for older people who are living with life limiting illness. Palliative care is defined by the World Health Organization (WHO) as an approach that: "…improves the quality of life of patients and their families facing problems associated with life-threatening illness, through the prevention and relief of suffering by means of early identification and impeccable assessment and treatment of pain and other problems, physical, psychosocial and social" (World Health Organization, 2010).

2.2 A Brief History of Palliative Care

Palliative care is a young discipline, emerging in the 1960s from the important work of key individuals who improved the care of dying people in societies where there was little provision for dying people (Clark, 2007). Palliative care (also known as 'Hospice care' in areas like North America) can be provided in different settings, such hospital, the community, home, and specialized inpatient units, also known as 'hospices' (Jordan et al., 2020). The modern hospice movement began in the 1960s in England, with the founding of St. Christopher's Hospice in London by Dame Cicely Saunders (2001). Dame Cicely Saunders was a nurse and physician, who recognized the need for specialized care for terminally ill patients. She created a model of care that focused on managing pain and other symptoms, which provided emotional and spiritual support to improve the overall quality-of-life for patients and their families (Clark, 1998). Dame Cicely Saunders, and other hospice pioneers, used innovative technologies of the era to provide symptom focused care. For example, the development of the portable battery-operated continuous

A. C. Nwosu et al., *Technologies in Palliative Care for Older People*, Synthesis Lectures on Technology and Health, https://doi.org/10.1007/978-3-032-04277-4_2

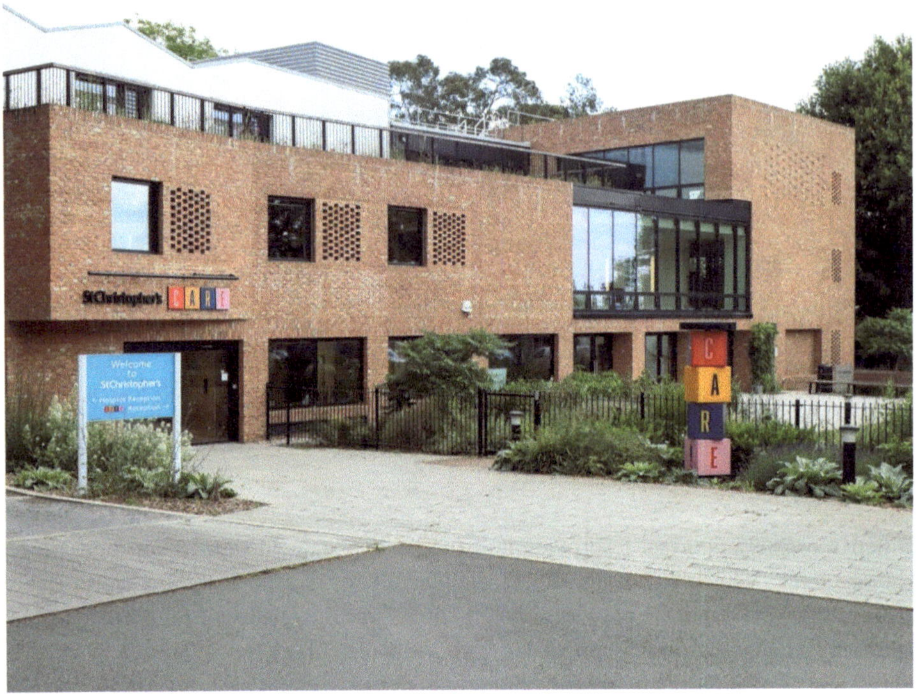

Fig. 2.1 St. Christopher's centre for awareness and response to end of life (CARE) as it is today, adjacent to the original St. Christopher's Hospice building. *Credit* St. Christopher's Hospice

subcutaneous infusion pump (known as a syringe driver) in 1979 by Dr Paul Russell has revolutionized medication delivery for pain and symptom management (Graham and Clark, 2005). Other examples include the use of tape recorders to capture patient views of their symptom control, when establishing the evidence for using opioids for cancer pain management, and the use of a hole punch card system (in the pre-computer era) to analyze symptom data of 1100 patients (Saunders, 2001). The hospice movement has since spread around the world, with hospices and palliative care services available in many countries (Clark, 1998) (Fig. 2.1).

2.3 Different Models of Palliative Care Delivery

Palliative care is delivered by multi-professional staff and services, across various settings, through different care models. These care models include:

- **Hospice care**, which focuses on providing individuals with personalized holistic management of their physical, psychological, social and spiritual care needs. Depending on the healthcare system, the term 'hospice' may describe a specialist inpatient facility (usually in a community setting, however in hospital services also exist) or describe the specialist palliative care provision delivered to a person in their home (Jordan et al., 2020).
- **Hospital-based care,** which is provided in a hospital setting, involving either a hospital-based palliative care team who support the patient's primary medical team to manage symptoms and improve quality-of-life, or an inpatient palliative care unit where the palliative care team provide direct care for patients (Hui and Bruera, 2020).
- **Community-based palliative care**, where holistic care is provided in the community by the family practitioner, district nurses and community palliative care specialists and other services, to support patients and families in their homes, nursing homes, or assisted-living facilities. The community-based palliative care team provides symptom management, emotional support, and coordinates care with other healthcare providers (Chan et al., 2021).
- **Integrated palliative care**, where palliative care is integrated into the primary medical care of patients with serious illnesses, through multidisciplinary partnership of care providers. A patient may receive palliative care services alongside other specialist interventions from community services and other specialist healthcare professionals. Examples include the management of people affected by chronic conditions, such as heart failure, chronic respiratory diseases and renal failure. The integrated palliative care team works with the patient's primary medical team to provide symptom management, emotional support, and to help coordinate care for the individual, depending on their needs and care setting (Bone et al., 2016).

2.4 Why is Palliative Care Important for Older People?

Palliative care is essential to improve quality of care for older people living with incurable disease and long-term health conditions (Burns, 2006). The importance of palliative care for older people is increasing due to growing global palliative need, which is a consequence of population aging (World Health Organization: regional office for Europe, 2011). Population aging is a global demographic trend where the proportion of older people increases while the younger population declines. This phenomenon is a consequence of declining birth rates and increased life expectancy in many countries, which is causing the working age population to shrink at the same time as an increasing number of older people require support (World Health Organization, 2024). Population aging causes the 'population pyramid' (which describes a graphical illustration of populations by age groups and sex) to appear "upside-down", due to increased numbers of older people plotted at the top of the pyramid (Fig. 2.2) (Roser, 2019). The 'upside down pyramid' poses several economic and social challenges, such as workforce shortages and increased health and social care needs of older people (Roser, 2019).

Older people are more likely to develop cancer, have several long-term health conditions (such as frailty) and develop dementia (Llop-Medina et al., 2022). Palliative care is an essential component of good care for everyone (irrespective of the cancer or non-cancer diagnosis), meaning that aging populations will increase their need for palliative care, as they develop age-related illnesses (Burns, 2006). Global palliative care need is expected to increase by 87% by 2060, with the increase primarily driven by the increase of palliative care need for people aged 70 or older (183% increase between 2016 and 2060) (Sleeman et al., 2019). Palliative care need is expected increase most rapidly for people with dementia, with global need expected to be 6 million people in 2060, a 264% increase between 2016 and 2060 (Sleeman et al., 2019). Older people, and their family caregivers, have several palliative care needs, which include emotional, physical, information, spiritual, social and financial (Llop-Medina et al., 2022). Consequently, it is important that world leaders recognize the needs of older people (and those important to them) to ensure that healthcare systems are equipped to provide the patient-focused approaches, that are necessary, to ensure that increasing numbers of older people are supported to live well until they die (Burns, 2006).

2.5 Challenges for Future Palliative Care Delivery for Older People

In the Western world the combination of various demographic, health-related and socio-economic factors will contribute to an increase in morbidity and mortality over the next decade (Etkind et al., 2017). On a societal level, there is a shift to patient choice, combined with increasing public awareness and dialogue about palliative care, and emphasis on personalized supportive care (Pemberton, 2013). Collectively, these issues provide challenges to future provision of global palliative care, which we illustrate below.

2.6 The Challenge of Providing Early Access to Palliative Care Services

Early access to palliative care services improves the quality-of-life for patients and their families; however, this can increase the work required from palliative care services, which increases pressure on a small workforce (Haun et al., 2017; Ahmedzai and Walsh, 2000). Initially, specialist palliative care services (encompassing all hospice and specialist palliative care services) were focused on cancer patients who were dying (Kaasa, 2013). However, as the range of treatments for cancer has increased, and palliative care has developed, many patients now may continue to receive active treatments as they approach

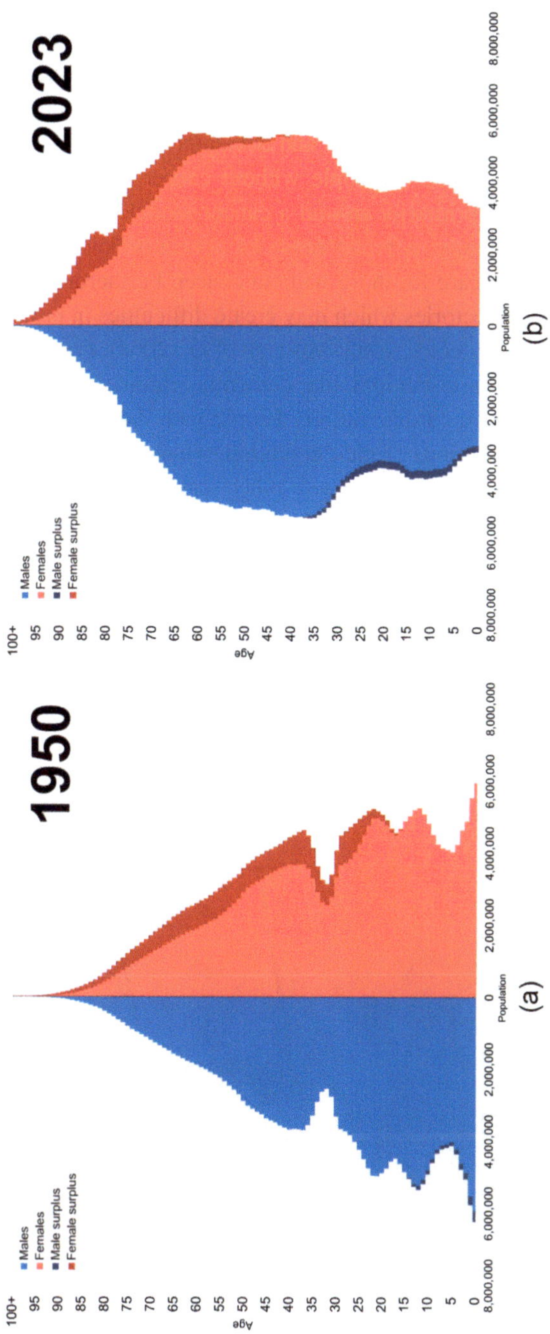

Fig. 2.2 **a** and **b**: Population Pyramid for the European Union, years 1950 and 2023. Tweedle, CC BY-SA 4.0, via Wikimedia commons

the dying phase of their illness (Addington-Hall, 2002). As palliative care became more established, decision makers argued that specialist palliative care should be needs-based, available to all (i.e., cancer and non-cancer) throughout illness (from diagnosis to death) and not restricted to end-of-life care (Ahmedzai and Walsh 2000; Department of Health, 2013). Consequently, palliative care services have expanded to include non-cancer illnesses; for example, older people with frailty and dementia (Addington-Hall et al., 1998). However, the palliative care needs of people without cancer may not be addressed by a healthcare system designed primarily around a cancer model (Fallon and Foley, 2012; Bone et al., 2017). Consequently, a broad range of specialist knowledge is needed to provide appropriate palliative care for those without cancer. Furthermore, non-cancer diseases have varying illness trajectories which may create difficulties in prognostication and advance care planning (Murray et al., 2005; Murtagh et al., 2004). For example, prognostication is often challenging in conditions like dementia, chronic obstructive pulmonary disease (COPD) and congestive cardiac failure. People with these (non cancer) illnesses may be prone to acute exacerbations of their condition, which may require active medical (or surgical) management and shared care with other services (Fallon and Foley, 2012). (Fig. 2.3).

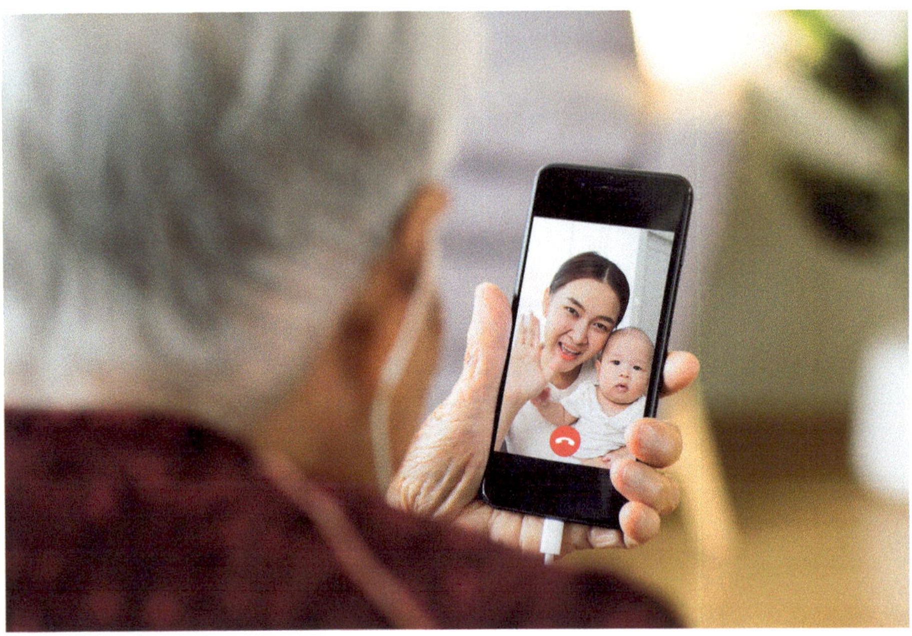

Fig. 2.3 *Credit* Nattakorn_Maneerat/Shutterstock

2.7 Challenges with Coordination of Palliative Care in Their Place of Care

Societies are aging worldwide, which is challenging for policymakers when determining how healthcare systems can best support older people requiring palliative care at home (Bone et al., 2017). Palliative care is delivered across several settings (e.g., hospice, community, and hospital) and the needs of patients (and the availability of services) is based on several factors. It is important that healthcare leaders understand the palliative care needs of their populations, so services can be designed to enable provision of palliative care for people in their place of care. Therefore, it is important that healthcare systems provide the multi-faceted care needed to address the palliative care needs of older people. Current challenges include communication difficulties across settings, which are exacerbated by poor interoperability in healthcare ICT systems, which create barriers to sharing healthcare information between healthcare professionals (Firth et al., 2025). Other challenges include difficulties in communication between multi-disciplinary team members, which can be further challenging in geographical remote areas with limited access to healthcare services (e.g., in rural communities) (Lynch, 2013). Therefore, it is important that healthcare leaders acknowledge the needs of their populations, and develop the necessary partnerships with stakeholders needed to deliver care (Sleeman et al., 2019; Firth et al., 2025).

2.8 Inequality of Access to Palliative Care Services

It is important to ensure equity of access to palliative care services wherever people receive care; however, older people may experience inequality due to several factors (Lau and O'Connor, 2012). Groups who are commonly underrepresented by healthcare (and palliative care) services include frail older people, resource poor individuals (and groups), ethnic minorities, minorities in gender identity and sexual orientation, rural (or isolated) communities and the homeless (Ahmed et al., 2004). Many people may experience inequality in receiving palliative care due to poor access to modern information and communications technology (ICT), that are increasingly required to access services. Consequently, services leaders need to ensure that innovations in AgeTech are used constructively to aim to improve access for users, rather than further exacerbating inequity (Lau and O'Connor, 2012).

2.9 Training Challenges for the Palliative Care Workforce

Healthcare systems need to deliver high-quality undergraduate and postgraduate training programs, to educate a muti-professional specialist and generalist workforce (Health Education England, 2014; Shape of Training independent review, 2013). However, common global challenges to palliative care training include poorly developed curriculum, lack of dedicated training, limited opportunities for clinical practice, lack of interdisciplinary learning, a focus on curative healthcare and a lack of recognition of the importance of palliative care (Aldridge et al., 2016).

2.10 Research Challenges in Palliative Care

Palliative and end-of-life care research receives less research funding than other disciplines, which limits the ability of researchers to generate the evidence needed to support healthcare organizations, and professionals, to deliver the best care for people and their families (Sleeman et al., 2012) (Fig. 2.4).

Palliative care research has infrastructural challenges, which add complexity to conducting research in older people. These challenges include governance issues, where

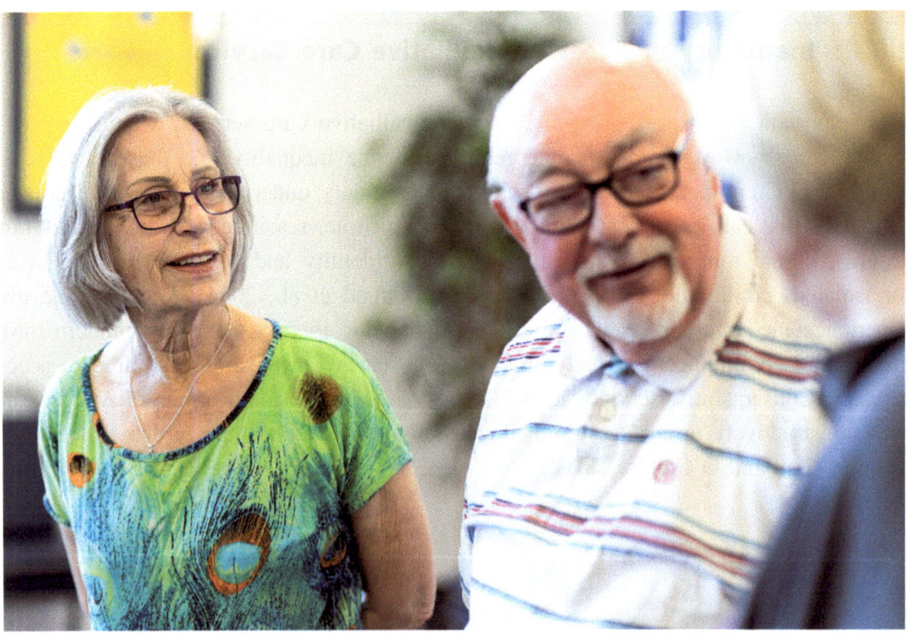

Fig. 2.4 *Credit* In-press photography/aging better

issues around legal indemnity and sponsorship can prevent the capacity for smaller palliative care organizations who lack this support (e.g., hospices) to participate in research.

Palliative care research studies have methodological challenges, as many studies are small, involving unwell people who are at risk of dying. Consequently, compared to other disciplines, palliative care research studies may recruit fewer people, who have greater risk of losing capacity to consent to research participation, and may die before the study ends. Furthermore, small studies may not generate the level of data needed to provide the evidence necessary to make recommendations about clinical practice.

Palliative care studies receive less support from the pharmaceutical industry, potentially due to the cost implications of developing new treatments for people with serious illness. Healthcare staff may exhibit 'gatekeeping' behaviors which may reduce opportunities for their patients to participate in research, due to unwarranted concerns that research participation is burdensome for palliative care patients (Higginson, 2016; Kars et al., 2016). However, research (exploring the preferences of palliative care patients) consistently illustrates the willingness of people with palliative needs to be involved in research (Nwosu et al., 2013; Chatland et al., 2023).

Compared to other disciplines, there is a shortage of palliative care researchers who can generate the evidence-based research required to improve care. This shortage is due to a variety of factors, including those described above, but is further complicated by palliative care originating external to traditional university structures, leading to under-representation of palliative care in academia (Higginson, 2016). AgeTech research has the potential to improve palliative care for older people; however, many research findings may not currently translate as many interventions lack evaluation for the specific needs of people with serious illness (Nwosu et al., 2022; Finucane et al., 2020). Therefore, researchers need to generate evidence to support the use of AgeTech in managing the palliative care needs of older people.

2.11 Find Out More

World Health Organization (WHO) Factsheet describing key facts about Palliative Care on a global level.

https://www.who.int/news-room/fact-sheets/detail/palliative-care.

The Center to Advance Palliative Care (CAPC).

CAPC is a national USA organization which is dedicated to increasing the availability of quality, equitable health care for people living with serious illness.

https://www.capc.org/.

Get Palliative Care.

Get Palliative Care is a public-facing website, provided by the USA Center to Advance Palliative Care (CAPC), which provides clear, comprehensive palliative care information for people living with a serious illness. Key features of the site include a Palliative Care Provider Directory, a definition of palliative care, and detailed descriptions of what palliative care does and how to get it.

https://getpalliativecare.org.

Editorial by Professor Irene Higginson describing research challenges in Palliative Care Research.

https://spcare.bmj.com/content/6/1/2.

References

Addington-hall, J., Fakhoury, W. & Mccarthy, M. 1998. Specialist palliative care in nonmalignant disease. *Palliative Medicine,* 12, 417–427.

Addington-hall, J. 2002. Research sensitivities to palliative care patients. *Eur J Cancer Care (Engl),* 11, 220–4.

Ahmed, N., Bestall, J. C., Ahmedzai, S. H., Payne, S. A., Clark, D. & Noble, B. 2004. Systematic review of the problems and issues of accessing specialist palliative care by patients, carers and health and social care professionals. *Palliat Med,* 18, 525–42.

Ahmedzai, S. H. & Walsh, D. 2000. Palliative medicine and modern cancer care. *Semin Oncol,* 27, 1-6.

Aldridge, M. D., Hasselaar, J., Garralda, E., van der Eerden, M., Stevenson, D., Mckendrick, K., Centeno, C. & Meier, D. E. 2016. Education, implementation, and policy barriers to greater integration of palliative care: a literature review. *Palliative medicine,* 30, 224–239.

Bone, A. E., Morgan, M., Maddocks, M., Sleeman, K. E., Wright, J., Taherzadeh, S., Ellis-smith, C., Higginson, I. J. & Evans, C. J. 2016. Developing a model of short-term integrated palliative and supportive care for frail older people in community settings: perspectives of older people, carers and other key stakeholders. *Age Ageing,* 45, 863–873.

Bone, A. E., Gomes, B., Etkind, S. N., Verne, J., Murtagh, F. E. M., Evans, C. J. & Higginson, I., J. 2017. What is the impact of population ageing on the future provision of end-of-life care? Population-based projections of place of death. *Palliative Medicine*, 32, 329–336.

Burns, E. 2006. *Palliative and End of Life Care of Older People*, British Geriatrics Society.

Chan, H. Y.-L., Chung, C. K.-M., Tam, S. S.-C. & Chow, R. S.-K. 2021. Community palliative care services on addressing physical and psychosocial needs in people with advanced illness: a prospective cohort study. *BMC Palliative Care,* 20, 1–8.

Chatland, L. E., Harvey, C., Kelly, K., Paradine, S., Bhagat, M. & Hudson, B. F. 2023. Research participation in palliative medicine—benefits and barriers for patients and families: rapid review and thematic synthesis. *BMJ Supportive & Palliative Care,* 13, 35–44.

Clark, D. 1998. Originating a movement: Cicely Saunders and the development of St Christopher's Hospice, 1957–1967. *Mortality,* 3, 43–63.

Clark, D. 2005. *Cicely Saunders: Founder of the hospice movement: Selected letters 1959–1999*, Oxford University Press, USA.

Clark, D. 2007. From margins to centre: a review of the history of palliative care in cancer. *Lancet Oncol,* 8, 430–8.

Clarke, D. 2013. *History of the Hospice movement* [Online]. Help the hospices. Available: http://www.helpthehospices.org.uk/media-centre/what-is-hospice-care/hospice-history/ [Accessed].

Department of health 2013. More care, less pathway: a review of the Liverpool Care Pathway.

Etkind, S. N., Bone, A. E., Gomes, B., Lovell, N., Evans, C. J., Higginson, I. J. & Murtagh, F. E. M. 2017. How many people will need palliative care in 2040? Past trends, future projections and implications for services. *BMC Medicine,* 15, 102.

Fallon, M. & Foley, P. 2012. Rising to the challenge of palliative care for non-malignant disease. *Palliat Med,* 26, 99–100.

Finucane, A., O'donnell, H., Lugton, J., Swenson, C. & Pagliari, C. 2020. Digital Health Interventions in Palliative Care: A Systematic Meta-Review and Evidence Synthesis. *medRxiv,* 2020.09.16.20195834.

Firth, A. M., Goodrich, J., Gaczkowska, I., Harding, R., Murtagh, F. E. & Evans, C. J. 2025. Community out-of-hours palliative care–'It'sa patchwork of services': A qualitative study exploring care provision. *Palliative Medicine,* 39, 245–255.

Graham, F. & Clark, D. 2005. The syringe driver and the subcutaneous route in palliative care: the inventor, the history and the implications. *Journal of pain and symptom management,* 29, 32–40.

Haun, M. W., Estel, S., Rücker, G., Friederich, H. C., Villalobos, M., Thomas, M. & Hartmann, M. 2017. Early palliative care for adults with advanced cancer. *Cochrane Database of Systematic Reviews.*

Health Education England 2014. Framework 15 | Health Education England Strategic Framework 2014–29.

Higginson, I. J. 2016. Research challenges in palliative and end of life care. *BMJ Supportive and Palliative Care,* 6, 2–4.

Hui, D. & Bruera, E. 2020. Models of Palliative Care Delivery for Patients With Cancer. *J Clin Oncol,* 38, 852–865.

Jordan, R. I., Allsop, M. J., Elmokhallalati, Y., Jackson, C. E., Edwards, H. L., Chapman, E. J., Deliens, L. & Bennett, M. I. 2020. Duration of palliative care before death in international routine practice: a systematic review and meta-analysis. *BMC medicine,* 18, 1–25.

Kaasa, S. 2013. Integration of general oncology and palliative care. *Lancet Oncol,* 14, 571–2.

Kars, M. C., van Thiel, G. J., van der Graaf, R., Moors, M., de Graeff, A. & van Delden, J. J. 2016. A systematic review of reasons for gatekeeping in palliative care research. *Palliative medicine,* 30, 533–548.

Lau, R. & O'connor, M. 2012. Behind the rhetoric: is palliative care equitably available for all? *Contemp Nurse,* 43, 56–63.

Llop-Medina, L., Fu, Y., Garcés-Ferrer, J. & Doñate-Martínez, A. 2022. Palliative care in older people with multimorbidities: a scoping review on the palliative care needs of patients, carers, and health professionals. *International journal of environmental research and public health,* 19, 3195.

Lynch, S. 2013. Hospice and palliative care access issues in rural areas. *American Journal of Hospice and Palliative Medicine®,* 30, 172–177.

Murray, S. A., Kendall, M., Boyd, K. & Sheikh, A. 2005. Illness trajectories and palliative care. *BMJ,* 330, 1007–1011.

Murtagh, F. E., Preston, M. & Higginson, I. 2004. Patterns of dying: palliative care for non-malignant disease. *Clin Med,* 4, 39–44.

Nwosu, A. C., Mcglinchey, T., Sanders, J., Stanley, S., Palfrey, J., Lubbers, P., Chapman, L., Finucane, A. & Mason, S. 2022. Identification of digital health priorities for palliative care research: modified delphi study. *JMIR aging,* 5, e32075.

Nwosu, A. C., Mayland, C. R., Mason, S., Varro, A. & Ellershaw, J. E. 2013. Patients want to be involved in end-of-life care research. *BMJ Supportive & Palliative Care.*

Pemberton, M. 2013. The Liverpool Care Pathway to dignity in death. Available: http://www.telegraph.co.uk/health/elderhealth/9796968/The-Liverpool-Care-Pathway-to-dignity-in-death.html [Accessed 14/08/2013].

Roser, M. 2019. The global population pyramid: How global demography has changed and what we can expect for the 21st century. *Our world in data.*

Saunders, C. 2001. The evolution of palliative care. *Journal of the royal society of medicine,* 94, 430–432.

Shape of Training Independent Review 2013. Shape of training: securing the future of excellent patient care. *In:* Professor David Greenaway (ed.).

Sixsmith, A. 2021. AgeTech: Technology-based solutions for aging societies. *Promoting the health of older adults: the Canadian experience,* 135.

Sleeman, K. E., Gomes, B. & Higginson, I. J. 2012. Research into end-of-life cancer care--investment is needed. *Lancet,* 379, 519.

Sleeman, K. E., de Brito, M., Etkind, S., Nkhoma, K., Guo, P., Higginson, I. J., Gomes, B. & Harding, R. 2019. The escalating global burden of serious health-related suffering: projections to 2060 by world regions, age groups, and health conditions. *The Lancet Global Health,* 7**,** e883–e892.

World Health Organization. 2024. *Ageing and health* [Online]. Website of the World Health Organization. Available: https://www.who.int/news-room/fact-sheets/detail/ageing-and-health [Accessed 24th March 2025].

World Health Organization. 2010. WHO Definition of Palliative Care [Online]. Available: http://www.who.int/cancer/palliative/definition/en/ [Accessed].

World Health Organization: Regional Office for Europe 2011. Palliative care for older people: better practices.

3 Digital Health and Palliative Care

3.1 The Challenge

This chapter provides a broad overview of emerging AgeTech, which can potentially to support the palliative care needs of older adults. In this chapter, we introduce AgeTech technologies that the reader will encounter in this book. The subsequent chapters are based on personas, focusing on the palliative care needs of the older person, and reference the AgeTech we introduce in this chapter.

3.2 Potential Use of AgeTech in Palliative Care

Digital health is defined as technologies which use computing platforms, connectivity, software, and sensors for health care and related purposes. Currently, AgeTech mostly facilitates early diagnosis and management of disease, supporting individuals to maintain their independence, and providing options for self-treatment of disease (Sixsmith, 2021). Global palliative care need is expected to increase due to several reasons, such as the socioeconomic consequences of an aging population. Therefore, it is important that healthcare leaders explore opportunities to use innovative technologies to help an increasingly frail and older population to access palliative care services (Bone et al., 2017). Digital health has been used to transform the delivery of health and social care, and help citizens to manage their own health (Topol, 2019; Department of Health Social Care, 2018; Haghi et al., 2017). Research demonstrates that digital health can improve delivery and access of healthcare services when used well. However, there is a lack of evidence about digital health research priorities in palliative care. Furthermore, many barriers limit the meaningful use of AgeTech in palliative care (Nwosu et al., 2018). These barriers include expense, interoperability, data privacy, security concerns, limited evidence, equity,

A. C. Nwosu et al., *Technologies in Palliative Care for Older People*, Synthesis Lectures on Technology and Health, https://doi.org/10.1007/978-3-032-04277-4_3

and the concern that technology will reduce face-to-face consults between patients and clinicians (Hancock et al., 2019; Nwosu et al., 2019). Improving the use of digital health in palliative has great potential to improve care delivery for many people with life-limiting illness (Nwosu et al., 2022).

The potential for AgeTech to support the evolving palliative care needs of older people has not been fully researched, meaning that many of the current AgeTech innovations may not address the needs of people with palliative care needs (Nwosu, 2023). There is also limited consensus about the AgeTech research priorities for older people with palliative care needs, and limited understanding of how AgeTech will improve care (Nwosu et al., 2022). It is important to prioritise the person-centered needs of users to identify how AgeTech can support their evolving care needs throughout illness. For example, the priority of an older person with new a diagnosis of cancer may initially be to receive information about the disease and to understand the treatment options. However, their needs may change as their condition develops, and they develop physical and symptom needs (which may require input by healthcare professionals and other service). Some people may have mobility and practical needs, which may require therapy services mobility aids, home modifications, practical assistance and help with transportation. Individuals may require other forms of support, such as companionship and assistance managing their estate and assets (physical and digital). AgeTech offers potential to support these needs, and many other palliative care needs, as people age. A brief overview of the different AgeTech technologies is presented next.

3.3 Artificial Intelligence Approaches (E.g., Machine Learning, Big Data, Natural Language Processing, Chatbots)

Artificial intelligence (AI) describes the science and engineering of developing intelligent machines, coordinated through algorithms or a set of rules, creating the ability of a machine to think and act like a human (McCarthy, 2004). AI involves different methodologies (e.g. machine learning, neural networks, deep learning, and natural language processing), which describes processes for a machine to be trained to act autonomously, with or without human instruction (Chen and Decary, 2020).

Artificial intelligence (AI) can be categorized into three main types: narrow AI, general AI, and super AI (Fjelland, 2020). Narrow AI (also known as weak AI) is used for specific tasks, such as voice assistants, recommendation systems, and self-driving cars. General AI (also known as strong AI) describes machines with human-level intelligence that can learn, reason, and solve problems in various areas. Super AI is a hypothetical stage of AI development where machines surpass human intelligence in all aspects (Genovese et al., 2024).

AI can be further classified into several types based on its applications and capabilities in disciplines, such as healthcare. Machine learning (ML) and deep learning AI analyze vast amounts of medical data to assist in diagnosis, treatment planning, and personalized medicine (Chen and Decary, 2020). Natural language processing (NLP) helps interpret and extract data from medical records, research papers, and patient histories (Lee et al., 2021). Large Language Models (LLMs) are used to understand and generate human language, through training of large amounts of text data to recognize patterns and produce coherent, contextually relevant responses (Taubert et al., 2024). Robotic process automation (RPA) streamlines administrative tasks like scheduling, billing, and data entry, improving efficiency in healthcare management (Hofmann et al., 2020). Additionally, predictive analytics using AI can predict disease outbreaks, patient deterioration, and treatment outcomes, enabling proactive care (Alowais et al., 2023).

AI has usefulness in healthcare practice, by facilitating analysis of large quantities of data contained within electronic healthcare datasets, which can support data interpretation (Shukla Shubhendu and Vijay, 2013; Quinn et al., 2021; Bajwa et al., 2021). AI can support palliative care management of older people in several ways, for example, on a population, clinical, individual and educational levels (Nwosu et al., 2022). On a population level, AI has been used to evaluate patterns of disease and to identify the palliative care needs of a population, using regional data (e.g. local, national, international) to identify trends of illness and recommend interventions. On a clinical level, AI has been used to predict survival of patients, using hospital electronic healthcare records, to classify pain severity, identify quality indicators, and identify serious illness conversations from electronic healthcare records (Einav et al., 2018; Makar et al., 2015; Sahni et al., 2018; Avati et al., 2018). On an individual level, AI has potential to use real-time data to facilitate personalized, palliative care, support for older people, according to their needs as they evolve, such as communication, treatment recommendations and companionship (Nwosu et al., 2018, 2019). In education, AI has the potential to support training for future palliative medicine doctors who will deliver care for older people with palliative care needs (Taubert et al., 2024).

AI is increasingly being used to preserve the memory of the dead, by creating a digital representation of a deceased person (an avatar). AI allows a living person to interact with the 'avatar' of a dead person. For example, an AI computer program (e.g., a chatbot) can be used to mimic the writing style of a dead person. Another example is the use of a computer to create a hologram of the deceased, to mimic their appearance, movements, and voice (Jiménez-Alonso and Brescó de Luna, 2023; Özdemir et al., 2021).

3.4 Mobile Devices, Wearables and Sensors

Mobile devices and wearables are used support palliative care in several ways, such as remote monitoring of physical activity and symptoms, delivery of well-being activities, documentation of advance care planning, for education, and access to policy and practice guidelines (Bienfait et al., 2020; Weekly et al., 2018; Meghani et al., 2017; Phongtankuel et al., 2018; Maggi et al., 2019). AgeTech can use these innovations to support palliative care of older people, by improving the capability of AgeTech devices to collect a variety of data (both health and non-health data) in combination with AI driven analysis and interpretation (Nwosu et al., 2018).

3.5 Telemedicine and Telecare

Telecare (describing the use of technology for personal alarms or monitoring systems, to support individuals), telehealth (a broader term, describing the use of technology to deliver healthcare services and information) and telemedicine (describing a subset of telehealth that focuses on clinical interactions and consultations conducted remotely) are increasingly used to provide palliative care provision for older adults (Wherton et al., 2020; Etkind et al., 2020; Hancock et al., 2019). Telehealth and telecare have been used to facilitate remote consultations between palliative care providers and patients (Bonsignore et al., 2018; Zeiser, 2023). These interventions may be useful where face-to-face visits are challenging, such as communities without access to specialist services (e.g. rural communities), people with mobility and/or transportation issues, and during public health emergencies (e.g. the COVID-19 pandemic) (Lally et al., 2021). Use of telehealth in palliative care is increasing and more research is needed to evaluate its usefulness in real-world settings (Hancock et al., 2019; Finucane et al., 2020) (Fig. 3.1).

Project ECHO (Extension for Community Healthcare Outcomes) is an example of a global tele-mentoring initiative, which is designed to create virtual communities of learners by bringing together healthcare providers and subject matter experts using videoconference technology, brief lecture presentations, and case-based learning, fostering an "all learn, all teach" approach (Manson et al., 2024; Project ECHO, 2025). Participants are engaged in the bi-directional virtual knowledge network by sharing clinical challenges and learning from experts and peers. Project ECHO has been recognized globally as a successful tool to improve patient care outcomes (Zhou et al., 2016; White et al., 2019). Unlike other telemedicine initiatives, Project ECHO focuses on development of learners, as opposed to fostering a relationship between healthcare provider and service users. Project ECHO is increasingly used to provide global support for hospices, staff and the wider palliative care sector. For example, Project ECHO forms a key part of national palliative care education strategies in Canada (Palliative Care ECHO Project - Pallidum Canada, 2025), the UK (Hospice UK, 2025) and Ireland (All Ireland Institute of Hospice and Palliative Care (AIIHPC), 2025).

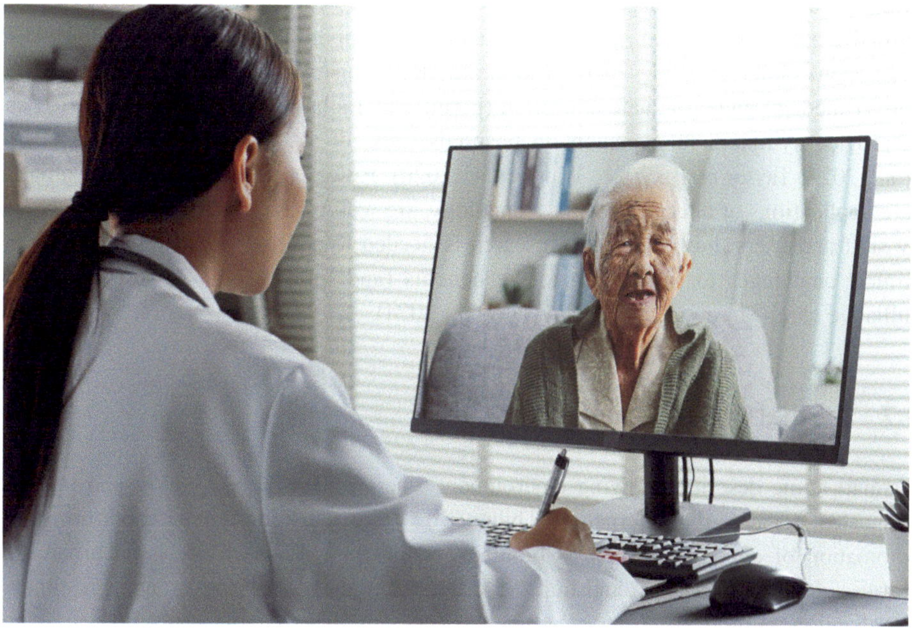

Fig. 3.1 *Credit* Nattakorn_Maneerat/Shutterstock

3.6 Alternate Realities: Virtual Reality, Augmented Reality, and Mixed Reality

Alternate reality technology describes the use of computerized technologies that use visual graphics, sounds and other sensory input to create an interactive computer world (Chirico et al., 2016). Alternate reality technology includes Virtual Reality (VR), Augmented Reality (AR) and Mixed Reality (MR). Alternate reality technologies are increasingly used in healthcare to enable the user to engage in three-dimensional experiences, using a headset (sometimes paired with handheld remotes) (Mo et al., 2022). VR is an entirely immersive process with a headset that covers the eyes and shuts out the external world, offering an immersive experience. Alternatively, AR uses technology to enhance the real-world environment of the user, by using technologies like smartphones, headsets, or digital glasses to project an image (or other digital information) onto their surroundings. With AR, the user is aware that they are still present in the real-world, with the AR supporting the user to interact with digital objects which are 'projected over' their physical space (e.g., the Pokémon Go video game) (Gerup et al., 2020). MR combines VR and AR, by merging the real world and digital objects into an interactive reality (Gerup et al., 2020).

Most alternate reality examples in healthcare involve VR, which is increasingly used to support care in different clinical scenarios, such as cancer care (Chirico et al., 2016;

Oyama et al., 2000) and surgery (Lee and Wong, 2019). VR is increasingly used to support palliative care (Martin et al., 2022), for example, to support advance care planning (ACP) discussions (Johnson et al., 2020; Niki et al., 2019; Austin et al., 2019; Hsieh, 2020), to deliver medical undergraduate education (Evans and Taubert, 2018; Lee et al., 2019) and to provide symptom management in hospitals (Niki et al., 2019) and hospices (Perna et al., 2021; Taylor et al., 2021; Wang et al., 2020). Research demonstrates that palliative care applications of alternate reality technology, are well tolerated and positively received by staff and users; however, more research is needed to address the methodological and clinical challenges to fully evaluate the benefits (and impact) of VR, AR and MR in palliative care (Mo et al., 2022; Nwosu et al., 2024).

3.7 Smart Homes and Cities

A smart home describes a living environment where sensor-based systems and internet-connected devices, the Internet of Things (IoT), are used for remote monitoring and automation of appliances, such as lighting and heating. A smart city is an urban area that uses IoT to collect data and improve city operations and services, such as healthcare coordination. (Liu et al., 2016). Researchers have published studies, which demonstrate how technology can support palliative care in situations where a patient's physical function is expected to decline (Pavic et al., 2020). Examples include voice recognition, chatbots, supportive robotics and IoT. It is increasingly important to develop the evidence-base to inform the meaningful use of smart homes (and smart city) infrastructure, which may potentially help to support the needs of an aging population, who will be living at home (many alone) with connected internet-enabled devices (Demiris and Hensel, 2009) (Fig. 3.2).

3.8 Robotics and Assistive Technologies

A robot is "a reprogrammable, multi-functional manipulator designed to move materials, parts, tools, or other specialized devices through various programmed motions for the performance of a variety of tasks" (Beasley, 2012). Robots are increasingly used for several clinical care applications (Beasley, 2012; Ceccarelli, 2011; Dallaway et al., 1995; Nwosu and Mason, 2012); for example, to conduct surgery (Roh et al., 2018), to deliver training (Randell et al., 2017; Pernar et al., 2017), to provide rehabilitation (Ona et al., 2018; Lefeber et al., 2017), for assistive personal care (Vandemeulebroucke et al., 2018; Bilyea et al., 2017), cleaning, automated medication delivery and equipment transportation (Beasley, 2012; Lavery et al., 2011). Robots have been used for assistive functions in dementia and elderly care (Martín et al., 2013; Darragh et al., 2017; Huschilt and Clune, 2012; Petersen et al., 2017). Therefore, robots can potentially support a variety

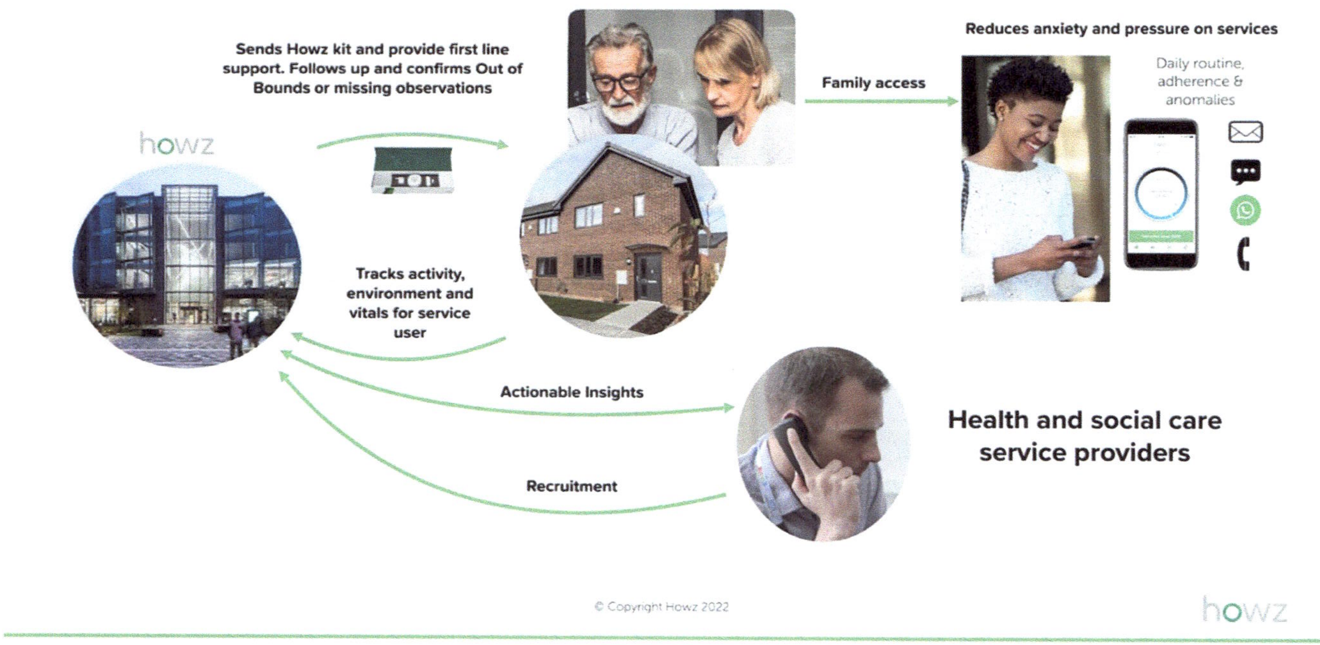

Fig. 3.2 Schematic demonstrating the interplay between the Howz sensor-based smart home set up for an older person living at home. This system consists involves data collection from sensors and household electricity usage, which informs data driven decision-making and communication with caregivers and healthcare providers. *Credit* HOWZ

of palliative care needs of older people; for example, by providing practical assistance, companionship, supporting mobility, and providing therapy (Nwosu et al., 2019).

3.9 Social Media

Social media are internet-based platforms that enable users to create and share content, build online communities, and interact with each other (Kaplan and Michael, 2010; Van de Belt et al., 2012). Examples (of an ever-increasing list of applications and platforms) include blogs, podcasts Instagram, Facebook, X (formerly Twitter), TikTok, Snapchat and many more. Online communities feature many discussions about palliative care topics, as these networks are increasingly used (by the public) to share information, connect and provide support (Taubert et al., 2014; Easwar et al., 2022) (Fig. 3.3).

Social media is increasingly used by public and professional stakeholders to share information about personal experiences of illness, death and bereavement (Taubert et al., 2014; Norris and Sofka, 2025). Social media has been used to raise societal awareness of palliative care issues, such as bereavement during the COVID-19 pandemic, thus creating opportunities to engage the public and facilitate stakeholder connection (Selman et al., 2021). Social media is increasingly used by healthcare professionals and policy makers;

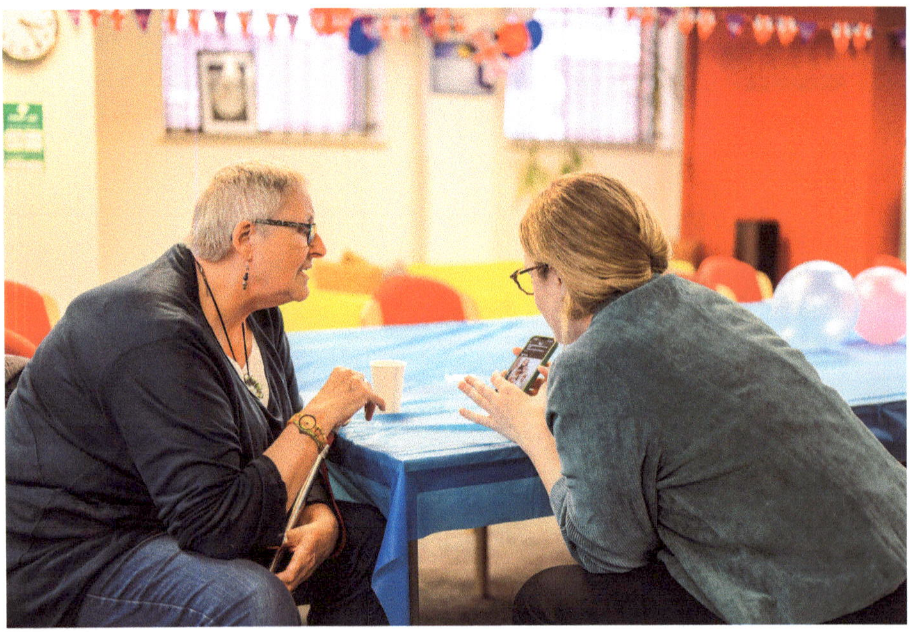

Fig. 3.3 *Credit* Carers centre tower hamlets/aging better

for example, to support service design and delivery, to engage with service users, for education and to conduct research (Nwosu et al., 2015; i Comabella and Wanat, 2015).

3.10 Digital Legacy

A digital legacy is the digital information that is available about someone following their death. Someone's digital legacy is often shaped by interactions the person made and information that they created before they died. This might include their social media profiles, online conversations, photos, videos, gaming profiles and their website or blog (The Digital Legacy Association, 2024). The volume of digital information generated by citizens is increasing, creating new opportunities and challenges after death (Taubert et al., 2014). There is potential to use technology to curate memories and preserve legacy; for example, users could prospectively, or retrospectively, use different forms of digital media to share memories of their own life (or the lives of those important to them) (Stanley et al., 2023). Digital legacy is increasingly important in society, with researchers and policymakers exploring how to support the public to manage digital information (belonging to them or those important to them) after death (e.g., personal data on social media networks) (Hayward and Martin, 2024).

Data stored on social media, cloud storage and other data networks can potentially be used to tell someone's life story, in ways not previously possible (Stanley et al., 2023). On a practical level, awareness of digital legacy is important for older people, as the current password and biometric restrictions of devices and data of accounts of deceased users, may create barriers for family and friends who wish to access this information after death. This creates practical challenges for bereaved families, who may be unable to access important information (e.g. financial information) and unable to access items with sentimental value (e.g. photos, videos, music) after the person's death (Coop and Marlow, 2019; Norris and Sofka, 2025). There are opportunities for health and social care professionals to include digital legacy planning as an emerging aspect of advance care planning (Norris, 2018), using support from organizations who are providing leadership in this area (e.g., the Digital Legacy Association—see Chap. 10 for more information) (The Digital Legacy Association, 2024; Norris and Sofka, 2025; The Digital Legacy Association, 2018; Norris et al., 2022; Norris et al., 2022).

3.11 Opportunities for AgeTech in Supporting Palliative Care Needs of Older People

AgeTech has the potential to improve choice and availability of palliative care services for older people, by creating new opportunities to deliver care, hence widening access to people unable to access face-to-face services. For example, AgeTech, integrated with face-to-face services, can potentially help healthcare providers to increase opportunities for users to access services, and enable providers to use resources more effectively. Communities in resource poor, rural or isolated areas may benefit from using AgeTech to remotely access to healthcare services, especially in situations where face-to-face support is challenging (e.g. due to geography, lack of resources etc. etc.) (Bonsignore et al., 2018). AgeTech can potentially improve the independence of older people with palliative care needs, by improving their ability to access information, contact healthcare professionals, record their treatment preferences, and self-manage their care needs (Petrova et al., 2018; Benze et al., 2019). There are opportunities to use the improving capabilities of AgeTech, combined with the increasing societal use of personal computing devices with data processing capabilities, to analyze users' data to personalize their healthcare.

3.12 Challenges of AgeTech Use in Supporting Palliative Care Needs of Older People

Challenges associated with AgeTech include governance issues about ensuring data privacy, security and accountability of users. It is important that AgeTech interventions are safe, evidence-based and are supported with a long-term strategy for its use, monitoring and evaluation (Topol, 2019). Long-term planning is challenging, due to the rapidly evolving nature of technology, and variation in how AgeTech applications are implemented, used and evaluated in different healthcare settings, services and economies. There is a risk of bias, if healthcare decisions are based on algorithms based on poor, or unrepresentative, data (The Academy of Medical Sciences, 2018). Consequently, there is a risk of increasing inequalities if AgeTech is not inclusive and accessible to some individuals (or groups), due to factors such as cost, geography, language, cultural factors, or disability (Phongtankuel et al., 2018). AgeTech may cause negative psychosocial changes in human interaction, towards machines and with other humans (Andtfolk et al., 2022). For example, there is potential that increasing use of AgeTech to provide clinical activity may contribute to a reduction in the number of face-to-face encounters between healthcare professionals and patients (Nwosu et al., 2017). Alternatively, AgeTech has the potential to improve healthcare access and choice for patients, especially for those who currently lack access to specialist palliative care services. In the digital age, society is currently experiencing the rise of AI generated 'virtual agents' (such as holograms, AI chatbots and avatars), which are digital human-like entities, specifically designed to elicit anthropomorphism from their owners and users (Koike and Loughnan, 2021). The use of the 'virtual agents' in AgeTech applications may cause users to anthropomorphize the technology, and develop emotional, and social, attachment, (Kühne and Peter, 2023). For example, users may develop emotional connection when interacting with smart devices and personal AI assistants and chatbots. Furthermore, users may use AI for companionship (for support during challenging times) to counter loneliness and for romantic relationships (Pan and Mou, 2024). People may use AgeTech for social relationships, which creates opportunities for exploration, experimentation and personal inquiry (Damiano and Dumouchel, 2018). However, the anthropomorphization of AgeTech creates practical, psychological and ethical challenges. For example, it is possible that emotional connections with AI may negatively affect human–human relationships, especially if the human users favor digital encounters over real-life relationships. Further, this technology may affect people's experience of grief, both for those who have physically died and virtual agents who 'die' digitally (i.e. deletion of data) (Figueroa-Torres, 2024; Banks, 2024). Consequently, AI offers several opportunities and challenges to shape human–human, and human–machine relationships, before and after death. The rapid development of AI therefore creates several cultural, ethical and legal issues, which we explore further in Chap. 10 in this book (Norris, 2024).

Poor or absent infrastructural, policy and governance structures will prevent healthcare services from successfully implementing, and providing, AgeTech in an coordinated and efficient way. It is important for organizations to develop (and adopt) appropriate models of care, to use AgeTech safely and effectively in clinical practice (Nwosu et al., 2022; Nwosu, 2023). For example, organizations require appropriate personnel and infrastructure to deliver AgeTech services, which may require long-term investment in equipment (e.g., servers), maintenance, upgrades and repairs. Without appropriate resources and planning, AgeTech may not be implemented in a meaningful, effective and cost-effective manner (Mandel et al., 2016).

AgeTech can be expensive for healthcare organizations to implement (Carr and Council, 2020). Notably, the costs of healthcare technologies are typically higher than consumer focused technologies; these high prices are further inflated by a lack of consumer demand for manufacturers to reduce AgeTech prices. The lack of consumer demand to lower prices is because AgeTech is used 'on' the consumer and not 'by' the consumer; however, in real world healthcare scenarios the 'consumer' is also the 'patient'. This is because the patient will pay for their healthcare (and the AgeTech product) either directly, or via insurance or taxes (Kumar, 2011). Although the patient (consumer) may pay for the product (to the manufacturer) and the service (to the health professionals), the demand is not created by the consumer. This may artificially create demand to justify the use of AgeTech, which increases costs to healthcare organizations and (hence) consumers (Kumar, 2011; Skinner, 2013). Costs to organizations are influenced by many factors, which require leaders to evaluate the specific merits of the options most suitable to meet the needs of the target population (Carr and Council, 2020). These evaluations may take time, and contribute to hidden fees for consultancy, testing, maintenance and technology upgrades, which increases expenses (ultimately for the patient) which may not have been initially considered (Kumar, 2011).

3.13 Brief Introduction to the Main Book Chapters

In the next chapters of this book, we further explore the possibilities of how technology can be used to support the palliative care needs of an older person, across different phases of their health trajectory (e.g., diagnosis, supportive care and end-of-life care). Our aim is to present the users' perspective of how AgeTech can potentially support palliative care in a speculative fashion, meaning our intention is to promote discussion, reflection and debate, as opposed to providing a detailed description of exactly how we imagine these technologies will (or should) be used in practice. We acknowledge that not all the innovations we describe in this book will be available to populations, due to many reasons such as practicality, availability, geography and usefulness. Equally, we acknowledge that due to the pace of innovation (for example, AI) it is inevitable that some AgeTech innovations will have developed further after the publication of this book.

We will reference the technologies introduced in this chapter, and we will further develop the ideas and themes, to discuss the opportunities and challenges of using these technologies in palliative care. In Chaps. 4–8 we focus on specific 'person-centered' topics where we focus on an individual with palliative care needs, and the potential benefit of using AgeTech in their lives. We will present the story from the perspective of an older person, by using 'personas' (semi-fictionalised case studies, based on quantitative and qualitative research, that are used to illustrate everyday experiences, problems and situations) to highlight how AgeTech technologies can offer 'real-world' support for the palliative care needs of people as they age. For each chapter, we initially present the 'challenge' to the individual regarding the chapter theme, followed by the persona and the potential AgeTech solution. The 'persona' chapters will address the opportunities and challenges of AgeTech in supporting the palliative care needs in older of people. The chapters will be structured around the following key challenge areas:

- Communication (Chap. 4)
- Physical health (Chap. 5)
- Psychosocial care (Chap. 6)
- Care coordination (Chap. 7)
- Care at the end-of-life (Chap. 8).

The focus of the book is how innovations in AgeTech affect individuals, as opposed to a detailed analysis of specific technologies. However, due to the continued development (and interest) in AI, we have provided one example in Chaps. 4–8 to illustrate how AI could potentially support palliative care. In Chap. 9, we focus on important issues related to AgeTech palliative care research, including challenges and priority areas for research. Chapter 10 summarises our findings, and discusses the emerging issues, limitations, important future directions, and the practical applications of palliative care AgeTech. This book will be of interest for healthcare practitioners, researchers, policymakers. After reading this book, the reader should:

- Understand the significance of palliative care needs of people as they age.
- Appreciate the potential of technology-based products and services to meet the needs of older people with palliative care needs.
- Develop understanding of the specific practical, research and policy challenges about the use of AgeTech in palliative care.
- Have greater insight of the main directions for research and innovation in these challenge areas.
- Understand some of the key policy and ethical challenges for AgeTech in palliative care.
- Understand good practice in working with people with palliative care needs.

3.14 Find Out More

Sheila Payne, Yakubu Salifu, Dunja Begovic, and Anthony Greenwood (eds.) The European MyPal study: Developing digital health for adults and children with cancer. ***Lancaster University (December 2022).***

https://mypal-project.eu/wp-content/uploads/MyPal-ebook-FINAL.pdf.

Artificial intelligence and new technologies in palliative care presentation by Dr Amara Nwosu at Hospice UK Conference—November 2023 (video and slide deck).

https://www.hospiceuk.org/publications-and-resources/artificial-intelligence-and-emerging-technologies.

Technology and future palliative care—Dr Amarachukwu Nwosu.

https://ehospice.com/editorial_posts/technology-and-future-palliative-care-dr-ami-nwosu/.

Jiménez-Alonso, B. and Brescó de Luna, I., 2023. Griefbots. A new way of communicating with the dead? Integrative Psychological and Behavioral Science, 57(2), pp.466–481.

https://doi.org/10.1007/s12124-022-09679-3.

References

All Ireland Institute of Hospice and Palliative Care (AIIHPC). 2025. *Project ECHO—All Ireland Institute of Hospice and Palliative Care (AIIHPC)* [Online]. Available: https://aiihpc.org/our_work/project-echo/ [Accessed].

Alowais, S. A., Alghamdi, S. S., Alsuhebany, N., Alqahtani, T., Alshaya, A. I., Almohareb, S. N., Aldairem, A., Alrashed, M., bin Saleh, K. & Badreldin, H. A. 2023. Revolutionizing healthcare: the role of artificial intelligence in clinical practice. *BMC medical education*, 23, 689.

Andtfolk, M., Nyholm, L., Eide, H. & Fagerström, L. 2022. Humanoid robots in the care of older persons: A scoping review. *Assistive Technology*, 34, 518–526.

AUSTIN, P., LOVELL, M. & SIDDALL, P. 2019. The Efficacy of Virtual Reality for Persistent Cancer Pain: A Call for Research. *J Pain Symptom Manage*, 58, e11–e14.

AVATI, A., JUNG, K., HARMAN, S., DOWNING, L., NG, A. & SHAH, N. H. 2018. Improving palliative care with deep learning. *BMC Med Inform Decis Mak*, 18, 122.

Bajwa, J., Munir, U., Nori, A. & Williams, B. 2021. Artificial intelligence in healthcare: transforming the practice of medicine. *Future Healthcare Journal,* 8, e188–e194.

Banks, J. 2024. Deletion, departure, death: Experiences of AI companion loss. *Journal of Social and Personal Relationships*, 41, 3547–3572.

Beasley, R. A. 2012. Medical Robots: Current Systems and Research Directions. *Journal of Robotics*, 2012, 14.

Benze, G., Nauck, F., Alt-Epping, B., Gianni, G., Bauknecht, T., Ettl, J., Munte, A., Kretzschmar, L. & Gaertner, J. 2019. PROutine: a feasibility study assessing surveillance of electronic patient reported outcomes and adherence via smartphone app in advanced cancer. *Ann Palliat Med*, 8, 104–111.

Bienfait, F., Petit, M., Pardenaud, R., Guineberteau, C. & Pignon, A. 2020. Applying M-Health to Palliative Care: A Systematic Review on the Use of M-Health in Monitoring Patients With Chronic Diseases and its Transposition in Palliative Care. *Am J Hosp Palliat Care*, 37, 549–564.

Bilyea, A., Seth, N., Nesathurai, S. & Abdullah, H. A. 2017. Robotic assistants in personal care: A scoping review. *Med Eng Phys*, 49, 1–6.

Bone, A. E., Gomes, B., Etkind, S. N., Verne, J., Murtagh, F. E. M., Evans, C. J. & Higginson, I., J. 2017. What is the impact of population ageing on the future provision of end-of-life care? Population-based projections of place of death. *Palliative Medicine*, 32, 329–336.

Bonsignore, L., Bloom, N., Steinhauser, K., Nichols, R., Allen, T., Twaddle, M. & Bull, J. 2018. Evaluating the feasibility and acceptability of a telehealth program in a rural palliative care population: TapCloud for palliative care. *Journal of pain and symptom management*, 56, 7–14.

Brinkman-Stoppelenburg, A., Rietjens, J. A. & van der Heide, A. 2014. The effects of advance care planning on end-of-life care: a systematic review. *Palliative medicine*, 28, 1000–1025.

Carr, A. & Council., F. F. 2020. The High Cost Of IT In Health Care. Available from: https://www.forbes.com/councils/forbesfinancecouncil/2020/01/02/the-high-cost-of-it-in-health-care/ [Accessed 29th November 2024].

Ceccarelli, M. 2011. Problems and issues for service robots in new applications. *International Journal of Social Robotics*, 3, 299–312.

Chan, A., Chien, I., Moseley, E., Salman, S., Kaminer Bourland, S., Lamas, D., Walling, A. M., Tulsky, J. A. & Lindvall, C. 2019. Deep learning algorithms to identify documentation of serious illness conversations during intensive care unit admissions. *Palliat Med*, 33, 187–196.

Chen, M. & Decary, M. 2020. Artificial intelligence in healthcare: An essential guide for health leaders. *Healthc Manage Forum*, 33, 10–18.

Chirico, A., Lucidi, F., de Laurentiis, M., Milanese, C., Napoli, A. & Giordano, A. 2016. Virtual Reality in Health System: Beyond Entertainment. A Mini-Review on the Efficacy of VR During Cancer Treatment. *J Cell Physiol*, 231, 275–87.

Coop, H. & Marlow, C. 2019. Do we prepare patients for their digital legacy? A survey of palliative care professionals. *Palliat Med*, 33, 114–115.

Copyright (c) Queen's Printer and Controller of HMSO 2017. This work was produced by Randell et al. under the terms of a commissioning contract issued by the Secretary of State for Health. This issue may be freely reproduced for the purposes of private research and study and extracts (or indeed, the full report) may be included in professional journals provided that suitable acknowledgement is made and the reproduction is not associated with any form of advertising. Applications for commercial reproduction should be addressed to: NIHR Journals Library, National Institute for Health Research, Evaluation, Trials and Studies Coordinating Centre, Alpha House, University of Southampton Science Park, Southampton SO16 7NS, UK.

Dallaway, J. L., Jackson, R. D. & Timmers, P. H. 1995. Rehabilitation robotics in Europe. *IEEE Transactions on rehabilitation engineering*, 3, 35–45.

Damiano, L. & Dumouchel, P. 2018. Anthropomorphism in human-robot co-evolution. Front Psychol, 9 (MAR), 1–9.

Darragh, M., Ahn, H. S., Macdonald, B., Liang, A., Peri, K., Kerse, N. & Broadbent, E. 2017. Homecare Robots to Improve Health and Well-Being in Mild Cognitive Impairment and Early Stage Dementia: Results From a Scoping Study. *J Am Med Dir Assoc*, 18, 1099.e1–1099.e4.

Demiris, G. & Hensel, B. 2009. "Smart homes" for patients at the end of life. *Journal of Housing for the Elderly*, 23, 106115.

Department of Health Social Care 2018. The future of healthcare: our vision for digital, data and technology in health and care. https://www.gov.uk/government/publications/the-future-of-healthcare-our-vision-for-digital-data-and-technology-in-health-and-care/the-future-of-healthcare-our-vision-for-digital-data-and-technology-in-health-and-care: DHSC London.

Easwar, S., Alonzi, S., Hirsch, J., Mossman, B. & Hoerger, M. 2022. Palliative Care TikTok: Describing the Landscape and Explaining Social Media Engagement. *Journal of Palliative Medicine*, 26, 360–365.

Einav, L., Finkelstein, A., Mullainathan, S. & Obermeyer, Z. 2018. Predictive modeling of U.S. health care spending in late life. *Science*, 360, 1462–1465.

Etkind, S. N., Bone, A. E., Lovell, N., Cripps, R. L., Harding, R., Higginson, I. J. & Sleeman, K. E. 2020. The Role and Response of Palliative Care and Hospice Services in Epidemics and Pandemics: A Rapid Review to Inform Practice During the COVID-19 Pandemic. *Journal of pain and symptom management*, 60, e31–e40.

Evans, L. & Taubert, M. 2018. State of the science: the doll is dead: simulation in palliative care education. *BMJ Support Palliat Care.*

Fallowfield, L. J., Jenkins, V. A. & Beveridge, H. A. 2002. Truth may hurt but deceit hurts more: communication in palliative care. *Palliative medicine*, 16, 297–303.

Figueroa-Torres, M. 2024. Affection as a service: Ghostbots and the changing nature of mourning. *Computer Law & Security Review*, 52, 105943.

Finucane, A., O'donnell, H., Lugton, J., Swenson, C. & Pagliari, C. 2020. Digital Health Interventions in Palliative Care: A Systematic Meta-Review and Evidence Synthesis. *medRxiv*, 2020.09.16.20195834.

Fjelland, R. 2020. Why general artificial intelligence will not be realized. *Humanities and Social Sciences Communications*, 7, 1–9.

Genovese, A., Borna, S., Gomez-Cabello, C. A., Haider, S. A., Prabha, S., Forte, A. J. & Veenstra, B. R. 2024. Artificial intelligence in clinical settings: a systematic review of its role in language translation and interpretation. *Annals of Translational Medicine*, 12, 117.

Gerup, J., Soerensen, C. B. & Dieckmann, P. 2020. Augmented reality and mixed reality for healthcare education beyond surgery: an integrative review. *International journal of medical education*, 11, 1.

Haghi, M., Thurow, K. & Stoll, R. 2017. Wearable Devices in Medical Internet of Things: Scientific Research and Commercially Available Devices. *Healthc Inform Res*, 23, 4–15.

Hancock, S., Preston, N., Jones, H. & Gadoud, A. 2019. Telehealth in palliative care is being described but not evaluated: a systematic review. *BMC Palliative Care*, 18, 114.

Hayward, S. & Martin, E. 2024. What you need to know about your digital legacy. *Good Housekeeping.*

Heintzelman, N. H., Taylor, R. J., Simonsen, L., Lustig, R., Anderko, D., Haythornthwaite, J. A., Childs, L. C. & Bova, G. S. 2013. Longitudinal analysis of pain in patients with metastatic prostate cancer using natural language processing of medical record text. *J Am Med Inform Assoc*, 20, 898–905.

Hofmann, P., Samp, C. & Urbach, N. 2020. Robotic process automation. *Electronic markets*, 30, 99–106.

Hospice UK. 2025. *Project ECHO* [Online]. Available: https://www.hospiceuk.org/innovation-hub/support-for-your-role/networks-communities/project-echo [Accessed].

Hsieh, W.-T. 2020. Virtual reality video promotes effectiveness in advance care planning. *BMC Palliative Care*, 19, 1–10.

Huschilt, J. & Clune, L. 2012. The use of socially assistive robots for dementia care. *J Gerontol Nurs*, 38, 15–9.

I Comabella, C. C. & Wanat, M. 2015. Using social media in supportive and palliative care research. *BMJ supportive & palliative care*, 5, 138–145.

Jiménez-Alonso, B. & Brescó de Luna, I. 2023. Griefbots. A new way of communicating with the dead? *Integrative Psychological and Behavioral Science*, 57, 466–481.

Johnson, T., Bauler, L., Vos, D., Hifko, A., Garg, P., Ahmed, M. & Raphelson, M. 2020. Virtual Reality Use for Symptom Management in Palliative Care: A Pilot Study to Assess User Perceptions. *Journal of Palliative Medicine.*

Kaplan, A. M. H., Michael. 2010. Users of the world, unite! The challenges and opportunities of Social Media. *Business Horizons*, 53, 10.

Koike, M. & Loughnan, S. 2021. Virtual relationships: Anthropomorphism in the digital age. *Social and Personality Psychology Compass*, 15, e12603.

Kühne, R. & Peter, J. 2023. Anthropomorphism in human–robot interactions: a multidimensional conceptualization. *Communication Theory*, 33, 42–52.

Kumar, R. K. 2011. Technology and healthcare costs. *Annals of pediatric cardiology*, 4, 84–86.

Lally, K., Kematick, B. S., Gorman, D. & Tulsky, J. 2021. Rapid Conversion of a Palliative Care Outpatient Clinic to Telehealth. *JCO Oncol Pract*, 17, e62–e67.

Lavery, H., Samadi, D. & Levinson, A. 2011. Not a zero-sum game: the adoption of robotics has increased overall prostatectomy utilization in the United States. *The Journal of Urology*, 185, e33.

Lee, A. L., Debest, M., Koeniger-Donohue, R., Strowman, S. R. & Mitchell, S. E. 2019. The feasibility and acceptability of using virtual world technology for interprofessional education in palliative care: a mixed methods study. *J Interprof Care*, 1–11.

Lee, R. Y., Brumback, L. C., Lober, W. B., Sibley, J., Nielsen, E. L., Treece, P. D., Kross, E. K., Loggers, E. T., Fausto, J. A. & Lindvall, C. 2021. Identifying goals of care conversations in the electronic health record using natural language processing and machine learning. *Journal of pain and symptom management*, 61, 136–142. e2.

Lee, C. & Wong, G. K. C. 2019. Virtual reality and augmented reality in the management of intracranial tumors: a review. *Journal of Clinical Neuroscience*, 62, 14–20.

Lefeber, N., Swinnen, E. & Kerckhofs, E. 2017. The immediate effects of robot-assistance on energy consumption and cardiorespiratory load during walking compared to walking without robot-assistance: a systematic review. *Disabil Rehabil Assist Technol*, 12, 657–671.

Lindvall, C., Lilley, E. J., Zupanc, S. N., Chien, I., Udelsman, B. V., Walling, A., Cooper, Z. & Tulsky, J. A. 2019. Natural Language Processing to Assess End-of-Life Quality Indicators in Cancer Patients Receiving Palliative Surgery. *J Palliat Med*, 22, 183–187.

Liu, L., Stroulia, E., Nikolaidis, I., Miguel-Cruz, A. & Rios Rincon, A. 2016. Smart homes and home health monitoring technologies for older adults: A systematic review. *Int J Med Inform*, 91, 44–59.

Lodhi, M. K., Ansari, R., Yao, Y., Keenan, G. M., Wilkie, D. J. & Khokhar, A. A. 2015a. Predictive Modeling for Comfortable Death Outcome Using Electronic Health Records. *Proc IEEE Int Congr Big Data*, 2015, 409–415.

Lodhi, M. K., Stifter, J., Yao, Y., Ansari, R., Kee-Nan, G. M., Wilkie, D. J. & Khokhar, A. A. 2015b. Predictive Modeling for End-of-Life Pain Outcome using Electronic Health Records. Adv Data Min, 9165, 56–68.

Maggi, N., Douglas Magnoni, L., Ruggiero, C., Gazzarata, R. & Giacomini, M. 2019. Information Technology System Including Patient Generated Health Data for Cancer Clinical Care and Research. *Stud Health Technol Inform*, 261, 289–293.

Makar, M., Ghassemi, M., Cutler, D. M. & Obermeyer, Z. 2015. Short-term Mortality Prediction for Elderly Patients Using Medicare Claims Data. *Int J Mach Learn Comput*, 5, 192–197.

Mandel, J. C., Kreda, D. A., Mandl, K. D., Kohane, I. S. & Ramoni, R. B. 2016. SMART on FHIR: a standards-based, interoperable apps platform for electronic health records. *J Am Med Inform Assoc*, 23, 899–908.

Manson, J., Gardiner, C., Taylor, P., Ghasemi, L., Westerdale-Shaw, E., Sutton, L. & Cawley, H. 2024. 'Palliative care education in nursing homes: a qualitative evaluation of telementoring. *BMJ Supportive & Palliative Care*, 14, e2147–e2153.

Martín, F., Agüero, C., Cañas, J. M., Abella, G., Benítez, R., Rivero, S., Valenti, M. & Martínez-Martín, P. 2013. Robots in therapy for dementia patients. *Journal of Physical Agents*, 7, 48–55.

Martin, J. L., Saredakis, D., Hutchinson, A. D., Crawford, G. B. & Loetscher, T. 2022. Virtual Reality in Palliative Care: A Systematic Review. *Healthcare (Basel)*, 10.

Mccarthy, J. 2004. What is artificial intelligence?

Meghani, S. H., Mackenzie, M. A., Morgan, B., Kang, Y., Wasim, A. & Sayani, S. 2017. Clinician-Targeted Mobile Apps in Palliative Care: A Systematic Review. *J Palliat Med*, 20, 1139–1147.

Mo, J., Vickerstaff, V., Minton, O., Tavabie, S., Taubert, M., Stone, P. & White, N. 2022. How effective is virtual reality technology in palliative care? A systematic review and meta-analysis. *Palliat Med*, 36, 1047–1058.

Niki, K., Okamoto, Y., Maeda, I., Mori, I., Ishii, R., Matsuda, Y., Takagi, T. & Uejima, E. 2019. A Novel Palliative Care Approach Using Virtual Reality for Improving Various Symptoms of Terminal Cancer Patients: A Preliminary Prospective, Multicenter Study. *J Palliat Med*, 22, 702–707.

Norris, J. & Sofka, C. 2025. *Digital Death Report 2025—Digital Legacy Association* [Online]. Available: https://digitallegacyassociation.org/about/reports-2/ [Accessed].

Norris, J., Sofka, C. & Ging, T. 2022. *Why Digital Assets planning and Digital Legacy safeguarding should form a holistic approach to advance care planning* [Online]. Available: https://www.researchgate.net/publication/364209840_Why_Digital_Assets_planning_and_Digital_Legacy_safeguarding_should_form_a_holistic_approach_to_advance_care_planning [Accessed].

Norris, J. 2024. *P-138 Dying in today's digital world, societal and healthcare perspectives in 2024* [Online]. British Medical Journal Publishing Group. Available: https://spcare.bmj.com/content/14/Suppl_4/A62.1 [Accessed].

Norris, J. 2018. Your digital legacy: an emerging aspect of advance care planning. Available from: https://www.rcp.ac.uk/news-and-media/news-and-opinion/your-digital-legacy-an-emerging-aspect-of-advance-care-planning/.

Nwosu, A. C. & Mason, S. 2012. Palliative medicine and smartphones: an opportunity for innovation? *BMJ Support Palliat Care*, 2, 75–7.

Nwosu, A. C., Debattista, M., Rooney, C. & Mason, S. 2015. Social media and palliative medicine: a retrospective 2-year analysis of global Twitter data to evaluate the use of technology to communicate about issues at the end of life. *BMJ Support Palliat Care*, 5, 207–12.

Nwosu, A. C., Collins, B. & Mason, S. 2018. Big Data analysis to improve care for people living with serious illness: The potential to use new emerging technology in palliative care. *Palliative Medicine*, 32, 164–166.

Nwosu, A. C., Sturgeon, B., Mcglinchey, T., Goodwin, C. D., Behera, A., Mason, S., Stanley, S. & Payne, T. R. 2019. Robotic technology for palliative and supportive care: Strengths, weaknesses, opportunities and threats. *Palliat Med*, 33, 1106–1113.

Nwosu, A. C., Mcglinchey, T., Sanders, J., Stanley, S., Palfrey, J., Lubbers, P., Chapman, L., Finucane, A. & Mason, S. 2022. Identification of digital health priorities for palliative care research: modified delphi study. *JMIR aging*, 5, e32075.

Nwosu, A. C., Mills, M., Roughneen, S., Stanley, S., Chapman, L. & Mason, S. R. 2024. Virtual reality in specialist palliative care: a feasibility study to enable clinical practice adoption. *BMJ supportive & palliative care*, 14, 47–51.

Nwosu, A. C., Collins, B. & Mason, S. 2017. Big Data analysis to improve care for people living with serious illness: The potential to use new emerging technology in palliative care. *Palliat Med*, 269216317726250.

Nwosu, A. C. 2023. Telehealth requires improved evidence to achieve its full potential in palliative care. SAGE Publications Sage UK: London, England.

Ona, E. D., Cano-de la Cuerda, R., Sanchez-Herrera, P., Balaguer, C. & Jardon, A. 2018. A Review of Robotics in Neurorehabilitation: Towards an Automated Process for Upper Limb. *J Healthc Eng*, 2018, 9758939.

Oyama, H., Kaneda, M., Katsumata, N., Akechi, T. & Ohsuga, M. 2000. Using the bedside wellness system during chemotherapy decreases fatigue and emesis in cancer patients. *Journal of medical systems*, 24, 173–182.

Özdemir, V., Springer, S., Yıldırım, A., Biçer, Ş., Kendirci, A., Şardaş, S., Kılıç, H., Hekim, N., Kunej, T. & Arga, K. Y. 2021. Thanatechnology and the living dead: New concepts in digital transformation and human-computer interaction. *OMICS: A Journal of Integrative Biology*, 25, 401–407.

Palliative Care ECHO Project—Pallidum Canada. 2025. *Palliative Care ECHO Project—Pallidum Canada* [Online]. Available: https://www.echopalliative.com/ [Accessed].

Pan, S. & Mou, Y. 2024. Constructing the meaning of human–AI romantic relationships from the perspectives of users dating the social chatbot Replika. *Personal Relationships.*

Pavic, M., Klaas, V., Theile, G., Kraft, J., Tröster, G., Blum, D. & Guckenberger, M. 2020. Mobile Health Technologies for Continuous Monitoring of Cancer Patients in Palliative Care Aiming to Predict Health Status Deterioration: A Feasibility Study. *J Palliat Med*, 23, 678–685.

Perna, M., MSW, Letizia, Lund, S., White, N. & Minton, O. 2021. The potential of personalized virtual reality in palliative care: a feasibility trial. *American Journal of Hospice and Palliative Medicine®*, 38, 1488–1494.

Pernar, L. I. M., Robertson, F. C., Tavakkoli, A., Sheu, E. G., Brooks, D. C. & Smink, D. S. 2017. An appraisal of the learning curve in robotic general surgery. *Surg Endosc*, 31, 4583–4596.

Petersen, S., Houston, S., Qin, H., Tague, C. & Studley, J. 2017. The Utilization of Robotic Pets in Dementia Care. *J Alzheimers Dis*, 55, 569–574.

Petrova, M., Riley, J., Abel, J. & Barclay, S. 2018. Crash course in EPaCCS (Electronic Palliative Care Coordination Systems): 8 years of successes and failures in patient data sharing to learn from. *BMJ supportive & palliative care*, 8, 447–455.

Phongtankuel, V., Adelman, R. D. & Reid, M. C. 2018. Mobile health technology and home hospice care: promise and pitfalls. *Prog Palliat Care*, 26, 137–141.

PROJECT ECHO. 2025. *Website of Project ECHO* [Online]. Available: https://projectecho.unm.edu/ [Accessed 22nd January 2025].

Quinn, TP, Senadeera, M, Jacobs, S, Coghlan, S, Le, V. 2021. Trust and medical AI: the challenges we face and the expertise needed to overcome them. *Journal of the American Medical Informatics Association*, 28(4), 890–894.

Randell, R., Honey, S., Hindmarsh, J., Alvarado, N., Greenhalgh, J., Pearman, A., Long, A., Cope, A., Gill, A., Gardner, P., Kotze, A., Wilkinson, D., Jayne, D., Croft, J. & Dowding, D. 2017. Health Services and Delivery Research. *A realist process evaluation of robot-assisted surgery: integration into routine practice and impacts on communication, collaboration and decision-making*. Southampton (UK): NIHR Journals Library.

Roh, H. F., Nam, S. H. & Kim, J. M. 2018. Robot-assisted laparoscopic surgery versus conventional laparoscopic surgery in randomized controlled trials: A systematic review and meta-analysis. *PLoS One*, 13, e0191628.

Sahni, N., Simon, G. & Arora, R. 2018. Development and Validation of Machine Learning Models for Prediction of 1-Year Mortality Utilizing Electronic Medical Record Data Available at the End of Hospitalization in Multicondition Patients: a Proof-of-Concept Study. *J Gen Intern Med*, 33, 921–928.

Selman, L. E., Chamberlain, C., Sowden, R., Chao, D., Selman, D., Taubert, M. & Braude, P. 2021. Sadness, despair and anger when a patient dies alone from COVID-19: A thematic content analysis of Twitter data from bereaved family members and friends. *Palliat Med*, 2692163211017026.

Shukla Shubhendu S, Vijay J. 2013. Applicability of artificial intelligence in different fields of life. *International Journal of Scientific Engineering and Research*, 1(1), 28–35.

Sixsmith, A. 2021. AgeTech: Technology-based solutions for aging societies. *Promoting the health of older adults: the Canadian experience,* 135.

Skinner, J. S. 2013. The costly paradox of health-care technology. *MIT Tech Rev* http://www.technologyreview.com/news/518876/the-costly-paradox-of-healthcare-technology/. *Published September*, 5, 2013.

Stanley, S., Finucane, A., Thompson, A. & Nwosu, A. C. 2024. How can technology be used to support communication in palliative care beyond the covid-19 pandemic: a mixed-methods national survey of palliative care healthcare professionals. *BMC palliative care*, 23, 40.

Stanley, S., Higginbotham, K., Finucane, A. & Nwosu, A. C. 2023. A grounded theory study exploring palliative care healthcare professionals' experiences of managing digital legacy as part of advance care planning for people receiving palliative care. *Palliative Medicine*, 02692163231194198.

Taubert, M., Watts, G., Boland, J. & Radbruch, L. 2014. Palliative social media. *BMJ Supportive & Palliative Care*, 4, 13–18.

Taubert, M., Hackett, R. & Tavabie, S. 2024. Artificial intelligence and large language models in palliative medicine clinical practice and education. *BMJ Supportive & Palliative Care*, 15, 61–64.

Taylor, R., Norris, J., Mckay, P., West, C. & Wade, K. 2021. 'The room where it happens': An exploration of personalised virtual reality (VR)-bringing the home to the hospice during the covid-19 pandemic. *Palliative Medicine*, 120–120.

The Academy of Medical Sciences 2018. Our data-driven future in healthcare. Website of the Academy of Medical Sciences.

The Digital Legacy Association. 2018. Your digital legacy: an emerging aspect of advance care planning. Available from: https://www.rcp.ac.uk/news-and-media/news-and-opinion/your-digital-legacy-an-emerging-aspect-of-advance-care-planning/ [Accessed 16th March 2025].

The Digital Legacy Association. 2024. *The Digital Legacy Association* [Online]. The website of the Digital Legacy Association. Available: https://digitallegacyassociation.org/ [Accessed 2025].

Topol, E. 2019. Preparing the Healthcare Workforce to Deliver the Digital Future the Topol Review: An Independent Report on Behalf of the Secretary of State for Health and Social Care. *NHS Health Education: London, UK*.

van de Belt, T. H., Berben, S. A., Samsom, M., Engelen, L. J. & Schoonhoven, L. 2012. Use of social media by Western European hospitals: longitudinal study. *J Med Internet Res*, 14, e61.

Vandemeulebroucke, T., Dierckx DE Casterle, B. & Gastmans, C. 2018. The use of care robots in aged care: A systematic review of argument-based ethics literature. *Arch Gerontol Geriatr*, 74, 15–25.

Wang, S. S., Teo, W. Z., Teo, W. Z. & Chai, Y. W. 2020. Virtual reality as a bridge in palliative care during COVID-19. *Journal of palliative medicine*, 23, 756–756.

Weekly, T., Walker, N., Beck, J., Akers, S. & Weaver, M. 2018. A Review of Apps for Calming, Relaxation, and Mindfulness Interventions for Pediatric Palliative Care Patients. *Children (Basel)*, 5.

Wherton, J., Shaw, S., Papoutsi, C., Seuren, L. & Greenhalgh, T. 2020. Guidance on the introduction and use of video consultations during COVID-19: important lessons from qualitative research. *BMJ Leader*, leader-2020-000262.

White, C., Mcilfatrick, S., Dunwoody, L. & Watson, M. 2019. Supporting and improving community health services—a prospective evaluation of ECHO technology in community palliative care nursing teams. *BMJ supportive & palliative care*, 9, 202–208.

Zeiser, S. R. 2023. Quality Improvement Evaluation of a Veterans' Palliative Care Telehealth Music Therapy Program. *Music Therapy Perspectives*, 41, 54–62.

Zhou, C., Crawford, A., Serhal, E., Kurdyak, P. & Sockalingam, S. 2016. The impact of project ECHO on participant and patient outcomes: a systematic review. *Academic Medicine*, 91, 1439–1461.

Technology to Support Communication in Palliative Care Practice

4

4.1 The Challenge

Good communication is important to ensure that patients, and their caregivers, can share their preferences and wishes for treatment with healthcare professionals, to facilitate adequate care that aligns with their goals and preferences (Brinkman-Stoppelenburg et al., 2014; Fallowfield et al., 2002). Good communication between healthcare providers and patients is associated with positive outcomes, such as improved patient satisfaction, better achievement of patient identified goals and reduced caregiver burden (Engel et al., 2023). Palliative care communication is challenging, and research demonstrates that communication problems are the most common concern for patients receiving hospital care (O'Hara et al., 2018). New technologies offer opportunities to support communication (Stanley et al., 2024; Crosby et al., 2021), especially due to the continued integration of internet-enabled devices into daily life (The Academy of Medical Sciences, 2018). From a public perspective, the use of communication technologies (such as mobile phones, the Internet, social media, podcasts, video conferencing, streaming and others) are increasingly used to share information, stories and experiences (Bienfait et al., 2020). Healthcare professionals also use technologies to facilitate communication; for example, during the COVID-19 pandemic, many healthcare services used technologies to facilitate virtual communication and reduce the risk of viral transmission (Norris and Taubert, 2020). During the COVID-19 pandemic, palliative care teams worldwide used digital health tools to communicate within the Multidisciplinary Team to deliver education and to communicate with patients and family caregivers (Calton et al., 2020; Mackey et al., 2020). Consequently, it is important that healthcare providers consider the opportunities and challenges presented by technological developments in communication, to ensure these tools are used meaningfully in palliative care for older people (Stanley et al., 2024).

A. C. Nwosu et al., *Technologies in Palliative Care for Older People*, Synthesis Lectures on Technology and Health, https://doi.org/10.1007/978-3-032-04277-4_4

4.2 What's in This Chapter

This chapter discusses how technology can be used to support communication in the management of older people with palliative care needs. This chapter focuses on AgeTech applications, which describe opportunities to support communication between patients, caregivers, healthcare professionals and wider society. We use the persona of Carol to describe practical opportunities to use these technologies to support her palliative care needs as she lives with metastatic breast cancer. Carol's story outlines opportunities that arise from her use of technology, which provide her with practical support and empowerment. Also, we focus on potential applications of AgeTech to support communication in education, research, policy and public health. As communication is a unifying and important theme in healthcare, we hope that this chapter will interest practitioners and policy makers.

4.3 Persona and Scenario—Carol

Persona: Carol is a 66-year-old woman with a diagnosis of stage 4, metastatic breast cancer. Carol has breathlessness and fatigue due to cancer, which has limited her ability to socialize and communicate with others. Carol uses technology to help her to communicate with other people, to socialize, gather information and plan her care (Fig. 4.1).

Scenario: Carol grew up in Brazil and is a native Portuguese speaker. She moved to North London (UK) 15 years ago with her husband. Although Carol is highly proficient in English, she occasionally finds it difficult to follow some discussions when people talk quickly. Carol's husband died last year due to prostate cancer. Recently, Carol has been diagnosed with advanced breast cancer and has received palliative radiotherapy. Carol is breathless and fatigued; she uses portable oxygen throughout the day and uses walking aides to help her mobility. Carol has one son, Leo, who is in his 30's and lives in East London. Leo visits Carol after he finishes working at the weekend. Carol enjoys socializing with others, and she is excited when Leo visits. Most of Carol's close friends are in Brazil and she has a small number of close friends in London. Carol finds it difficult to make friends, due to her breathlessness and the language barrier. Leo is concerned that Carol is not communicating with other people throughout the day.

Solution: Leo encourages Carol to use technology to communicate with other people. Carol uses different social media platforms to communicate with her friends in Brazil. She uses the internet to gather information about her illness, including treatment options, survival rates and information to plan her funeral. Carol listens to podcasts to learn about people's experience of cancer, and she engages in online discussion forums (such as Reddit) to share her experience of living with cancer with other Portuguese speakers. Specifically, she uses these discussion groups to obtain information about the procedure

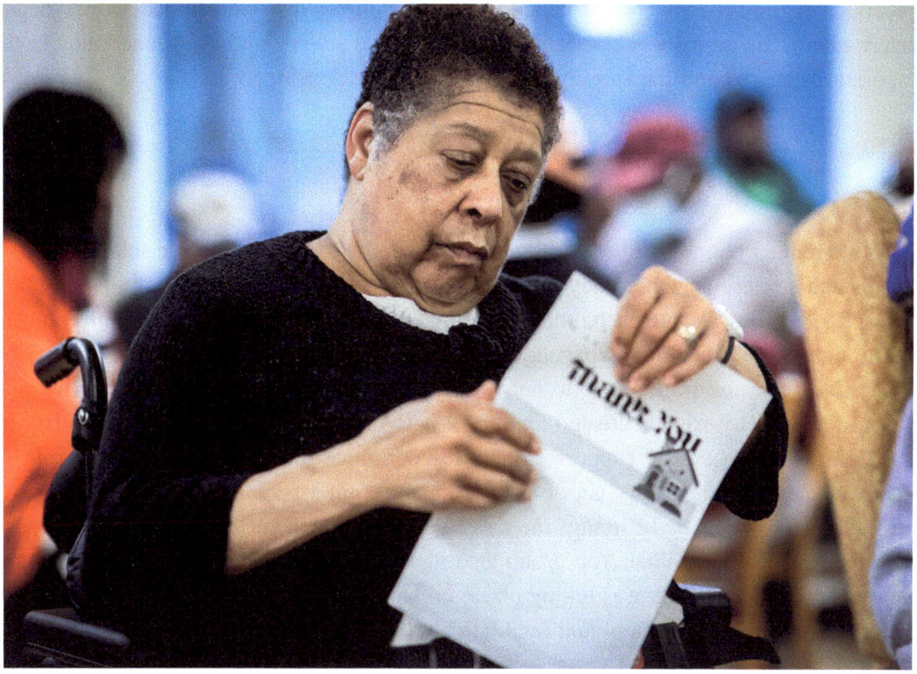

Fig. 4.1 *Credit* Independent age/aging better

required to arrange repatriation of her body to Brazil, for burial, following her death. She uses websites to document and organize her digital assets and record her wishes. She has also archived her important photos, videos and documents, which she has stored on an external hard drive and cloud storage for her son to access after her death.

4.4 Podcasts

Carol listened to several podcasts exploring the subject of breast cancer. She chose content which was related to her stage of disease. Some of the podcasts she listened to were in English, others were in Portuguese.

4.5 Social Media

Carol joined several Facebook groups for people diagnosed with breast cancer. She found the group informative and enjoyable; however, she found some of the content upsetting, as some of stories prompted her to think about her own illness and mortality. Carol used

Facebook to find a local breast cancer support group, which she joined as her health deteriorated. The group would meetup in person, once a week and she found value in the experiences shared and the subsequent friendships she developed.

4.6 Text Messaging Services

Carol shared her phone number with two group members, with whom she shared personal photos and stories. Together, they created a WhatsApp group, and they infrequently sent text and video messages to each other. They felt comfortable sharing personal information, due to their similar health and psychological journey.

As Carol became frailer (due to her illness), her friends travelled from Brazil to visit her in London. Her friends created another WhatsApp group (including her local friends and those from her cancer support groups) to coordinate practical support for Carol and Leo over the coming months. Carol arranged visits from a personal carer to help support her with activities of daily living; the carer was also added to the WhatsApp group by the group admin. The WhatsApp group also included Carol, and she was able to see the care and coordination that was taking place, on her (and Leo's) behalf. She was an active participant in the management and facilitation of her own care.

4.7 Online Tools to Document, and Organize, a Person's Digital Estate, Wishes and Memories

Carol was admitted to her local hospice a few months later. She hoped that her condition would improve. At this point in her journey, Carol had not made a Last Will & Testament to outline her wishes and preferences for what should happen with her possessions after her death. In the hospice, the doctor discussed a treatment escalation plan with Carol to plan her medical management; however, this plan did not include plans for her non-medical wishes (for example, planning around her digital estate and memories). Therefore, Carol used an online advance care planning (ACP) platform (MyWishes) to document and share her care preferences. She used MyWishes to write her 'Last Will & Testament', document her funeral wishes, record her ACP and document her wishes of how her online data should be managed after death (Fig. 4.2).

4.8 Digital Storage of Personal Photos and Videos

Most of Carol's photos were stored and saved on Facebook and Instagram. Carol believed that it was important that these photos and videos were not lost and will be available for her son. She downloaded an archive of her content from social media and provided copies

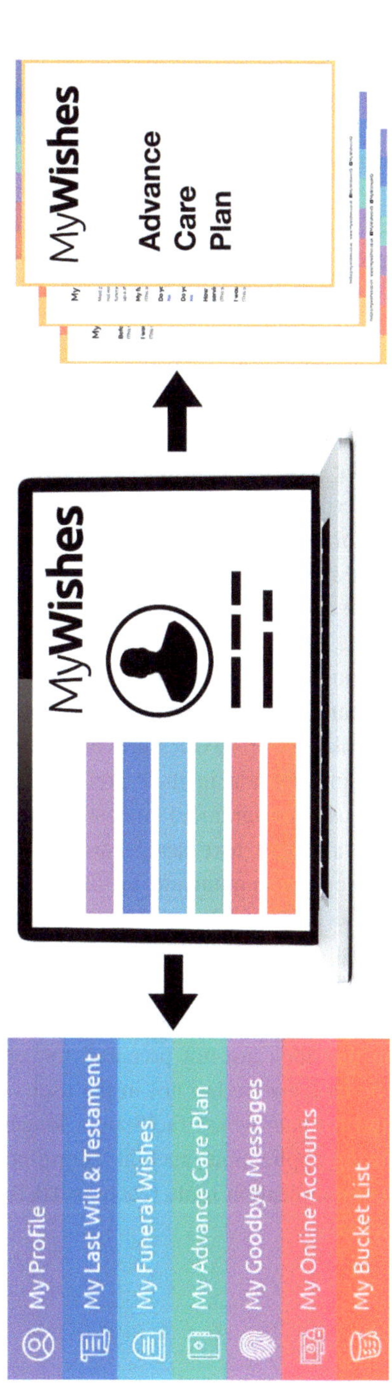

Fig. 4.2 MyWishes, an online tool to document, and organise, a person's digital estate, wishes and plans. (www.mywishes.co.uk/). *Credit* MyWishes

of the photos and video to family and friends on a portable memory flash drive. Carol decided to film a video message for her son that told him about her life. It included some memorable stories about, and she described her love for him. Carol used MyWishes to schedule a series of messages to be sent out on specific dates in the future. This included a message for Leo on his 40th Birthday.

4.9 Digital Communication Formats and Learning Styles

Technology has the potential to improve communication, by delivering content using the preferred learning style, or format, of the user. Educational theory suggests that individuals all have a particular approach, or style, of learning and that learning will be more effective, and efficient, if information is delivered according to their preferred learning style (Kolb, 2007). Different learning style models exists but examples includes the VARK model (Fleming, 2001), which describe how learners may prefer to learn through one or more modalities, including Visual (preference for information displayed as images or symbols), Aural (information that is *"heard or spoken")*, Read/write (information displayed as words), and Kinesthetic (experience and practice—simulated or real) (Drago and Wagner, 2004).

Technologies can support communication, according to learning styles. In healthcare, examples include blogs, podcasts and social media services like X (formerly Twitter), Threads, Snap, YouTube and TikTok. These services provide users (like Carol) with the opportunity to share, and receive information in their preferred format (Taubert et al., 2014). For example, a user may use Instagram to look at photos, YouTube to watch videos, and use a blog to obtain a longer text-based narrative on subject of interest. It is important to consider that people communicate in different ways and that digital methods of communication may be problematic in some situations. For example, it is possible that Carol may become distressed by viewing content which has been shared by other cancer patients on social media. Although Carol was able to use this experience positively, the experience may potentially be distressing for some people, especially if they are exposed to information that they are not prepared for, or do not want to see. Similarly, the information may be informative but not in the user's preferred format. For example, Carol may prefer digital formats which facilitate a longer, in-depth discussion about aspects of breast cancer, using applications such as Zoom, podcasts and long form blogs, compared to short-form communication tools (such as TikTok and X) which may not facilitate comprehensive discussion.

4.10 How Healthcare Providers Can Improve Digital Information for Palliative Care Service Users

The digital revolution, in combination with increased availability of online health literature, is empowering patients to learn more about their health (Kuwabara et al., 2020; Timmers et al., 2020). The availability of knowledge for the public is challenging to traditional medical epistemic authority structures (i.e. 'doctor knows best'), which placed medical professionals as expert judges of evidence-based medicine, responsible for medical decision-making (Popowicz, 2021). It is argued that the 'doctor knows best' model is becoming outdated and replaced with an 'empowered patient' model, which presents opportunities and challenges (Popowicz, 2021). The 'empowered patient' model potentially provides people with more, personalised information about their illness, which may facilitate deeper understanding of health, thus enabling the patient to make more informed choices about their care (Kuwabara et al., 2020). However, increased access to information increases the possibility that people will access spurious information, with unproven claims that can be misleading and potentially harmful, especially due the proliferation of commercially available AI health applications, which may not be subject to the conventional safety review and quality control processes (Zawati and Lang, 2024). Therefore, professional bodies and advocacy organizations have an important role in addressing the ethical and legal gaps in AgeTech applications, to ensure they are safe for users. Furthermore, it is important that healthcare providers carefully develop communication materials to meet the information needs of the users, by considering the structure and format of content, and learning style preferences of the user (Ishizumi et al., 2024; Fridman et al., 2023).

4.11 Opportunities to Use Technology to Support Communication in Palliative Care

There are opportunities for healthcare providers to explore how technologies can be used to support communication in palliative care. For example, there is potential to improve the use, and functionality, of messaging services (for example, text/short message service (SMS), email, images, video) to improve opportunities for patients to communicate with their healthcare team (Stanley et al., 2024; Dash et al., 2016). Websites of healthcare providers could be better designed, and updated, to provide more information about the services offered, and healthcare advice for patients and caregivers (Favela et al., 2004; Hamidi et al., 2019). Podcasts could be used by healthcare providers, caregivers and patients to share information about palliative care, and the experiences of service users (Nwosu et al., 2017). Chatbot technology (using NLP) could be used to help patients to obtain information (for example, from their medical record, the internet and from healthcare providers' websites) without needing to consult a human (for example, to find information about the opening hours and location hospital pharmacies in a geographical area) (Raza et al., 2022). Chatbots could be used by patients to contact a doctor to communicate information related to their disease (Greene et al., 2019). For example, Carol could use an AI voice assistant (e.g. Google Duplex) to autonomously make phone calls to her doctor to arrange face-to-face consultations (Matias and Leviathan, 2018). During the phone call, the chatbot could keep their place in the telephone queue, freeing Carol to do other things. When the healthcare professional answered the phone call, the chatbot could either answer on Carol's behalf or connect Carol to the call. Similarly, an AI chatbot could be used to exchange messages and images with Carol's healthcare team (Greene et al., 2019). Care providers could use digital tools to communicate wait times for appointments with their patients, which may be useful for people attending hospital appointments, as they could leave the waiting room (e.g., to have a drink in the cafeteria) and return to the clinic appointment when they receive an electronic notification on the phone which instructs them to return (Chakraborty et al., 2023).

4.12 Use of Social Media by Individuals and Groups to Raise Awareness of Palliative Care Issues

Social media can be used by individuals and groups to raise awareness about palliative care issues in society. Users may choose to use social media to provide a personal narrative of their experience, enabling others to provide comment and share their own story, on a wider (e.g., international) level. For example, Stephen Robert Sutton MBE (16 December 1994–14 May 2014), was an English blogger and charity activist known for his blog 'Stephen's Story', in addition to his fundraising efforts for the 'Teenage Cancer Trust' charity to help teenagers with cancer. By the second anniversary of his death, £5.5 million had been raised in his memory (BBC, 2016).

In the UK, officials have used social media, and the internet, to share public announcements about the health of the Royal Family (of the United Kingdom of Great Britain and Northern Ireland). Following the death of Queen Elizabeth II in 2022, the UK Government developed a website to coordinate the process for mourners to obtain a ticket to join a physical queue, to view the coffin of the deceased Monarch. The queue to view the coffin of Queen Elizabeth was miles long and had its own YouTube livestream (Sam Haysom, 2022). On 6th February 2024, Buckingham palace announced that King Charles the Third of the United Kingdom of Great Britain and Northern Ireland, was diagnosed with cancer. The Palace used its social media channels (X–formerly Twitter, and Instagram) to further share the news of the King's cancer diagnosis. Similarly, Catherine, Princess of Wales, released a video on the 22nd of March 2024 on Instagram, where she talked openly about her cancer diagnosis. In the video, Princess Catherine spoke about the major abdominal surgery she had received, the cancer diagnosis, her experience of chemotherapy, and the impact of the news on her family (Coughlan, 2025).

4.13 How Technology Can Support Communication in Compassionate Communities

Technology offers potential to support palliative care as part of the compassionate community movement, by improving connection between people, enabling coordination of support for seriously ill people in their communities (Abel and Taubert, 2020). 'Compassionate Communities' are networks of people supporting each other to live fully before they die (Kellehear, 2013). The aim of a 'Compassionate Community' is to help people to feel ready, willing, and confident to talk about death and dying and to be able to support each other in times of crisis and loss (Kellehear, 2013). The network can provide both hands-on care and support to carers (Abel, 2018). People within these communities can potentially use technologies to support the practical needs of older people. Apps can be useful to coordinate care needs. For example, the CareTeam app (http://careteam.club) provides a secure network to coordinate support for adults in their own homes, with the potential to include anyone involved in the care of an adult at home (e.g., family, friends, paid for care provision and healthcare professionals). The Jointly app (https://jointlyapp.com) is an app designed specifically for carers, which combines group messaging and to-do lists with other features, such as including medication lists and a shared calendar. Other apps provide a platform for people in communities to connect with each other, to better understand the needs of neighbors, share resources and skills and provide practical help. Examples include Favourhood (https://favourhood.app/), where neighbors will either ask for a favor, or offer a favor to others in their community (e.g., someone to do grocery shopping). Another example is Nextdoor (https://nextdoor.com/), a platform for neighbors to connect, exchange recommendations and offer other forms of practical support. People can also use app services to coordinate a cooking rota to plan meals for individuals and families, examples include MealTrain (https://www.mealtrain.com) and 'Take Them A Meal' (https://takethemameal.com/).

Healthcare professionals can build much stronger partnerships with these supportive networks and transform end-of-life care at home (Abel, 2018). Furthermore, international governments are increasingly recognizing the importance of community and social relationships for citizens, as strong social relationships are shown to reduce mortality, morbidity and reduce the financial cost of death and dying for the individual and for the state (Kellehear, 2020, Holt-Lunstad et al., 2010). Combined with 'smart city' approaches (an urban area that uses digital technology to collect data and operate services) for healthcare, there is an opportunity that AgeTech can improve palliative care by supporting the development of a 'smart city', 'compassionate community' model of care (Cook et al., 2018; Ahmad et al., 2022).

4.14 Artificial Intelligence Applications in Palliative Care Communication

AI is being used by practitioners to increase options for communication, for example, by providing information in a format and language preferable to users and creating potential for language translation services. A systematic review of AI medical translation, demonstrated that AI translation can potentially provide accurate translations for brief communications in limited languages; however, human translation is often necessary (Genovese et al., 2024). AI translation may be useful when a person's preferred language differs from the one used within the local health and social ecosystem. Commercially available AI translation services are available to the public, for example 'Mable Translate' is a smartphone app (on Apple and Android) which uses NLP to provide full voice-to-voice translation for medical translation (https://mabel.care) (Mabel AI, 2024; Rao et al., 2024; Sandhu et al., 2022).

4.15 Key Initiatives

Dr Kate Granger MBE FRCP (1981–2016) was an English geriatrician and campaigner, who used digital technologies, such as X (formally Twitter), to raise awareness about the impact of cancer on patients and families (Kate Granger, 2013). Dr Granger used her platform to engage with professionals, the media and the public to campaign about the importance of improving care (such as communication) for people living with serious illness. Dr Granger demonstrated that digital communication technologies used in a genuine and strategic way can act as a powerful tool to amplify a voice and a cause. Dr Granger was diagnosed with terminal sarcoma; she observed that doctors would often see her without introducing themselves. This experience led to Dr Granger, with her husband Chris, developing the 'Hello my name is…' campaign, with a simple message to encourage healthcare professionals to introduce themselves to their patients (Fig. 4.3).

> I made the stark observation that many staff looking after me did not introduce themselves before delivering my care. It felt incredibly wrong that such a basic step in communication was missing. After ranting at my husband during one evening's visiting time, he encouraged me to "stop whinging and do something!"—**Dr Kate Granger MBE FRCP** (Ban et al., 2021)

The 'Hello My Name Is…' campaign involved initiatives to raise awareness of the importance of communication with patients and caregivers (for example, the creation of 'Hello My Name Is…' name badges), and the delivery of communication training for healthcare staff. The campaign's momentum became an influential, social movement to internationally promote compassionate care (Topol, 2019).

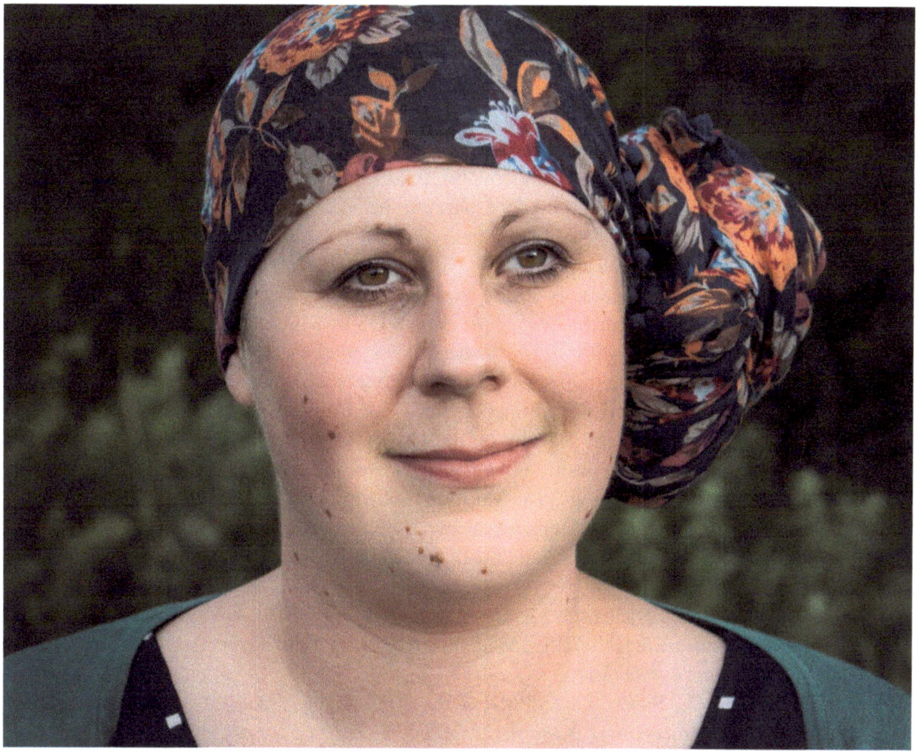

Fig. 4.3 Kate. *Credit* Chris Pointon

4.16 Find Out More

MyWishes Future Care Planning.

www.MyWishes.co.uk.

Hello My Name Is…

https://www.hellomynameis.org.uk.

Stephen Sutton.

https://www.teenagecancertrust.org/information-about-cancer/cancer-stories/stephen-sutton-mbe.

References

Abel, J. & Taubert, M. 2020. Coronavirus pandemic: compassionate communities and information technology. *BMJ Supportive & Palliative Care*, 10, 369–371.

Abel, J. 2018. Compassionate communities and end-of-life care. *Clinical Medicine*, 18, 6.

Ahmad, K. A. B., Khujamatov, H., Akhmedov, N., Bajuri, M. Y., Ahmad, M. N. & Ahmadian, A. 2022. Emerging trends and evolutions for smart city healthcare systems. *Sustainable Cities and Society*, 80, 103695.

Ban, S., Baker, K., Bradley, G., Derbyshire, J., Elliott, C., Haskin, M., Macknight, J. & Rosengarten, L. 2021. 'Hello, my name is…': an exploratory case study of inter-professional student experiences in practice. *British Journal of Nursing*, 30, 802–810.

BBC. 2016. *Stephen Sutton's legacy: £5.5m raised in his memory* [Online]. Website of the BBC. Available: https://www.bbc.co.uk/news/uk-england-stoke-staffordshire-36288677 [Accessed].

Bienfait, F., Petit, M., Pardenaud, R., Guineberteau, C. & Pignon, A. 2020. Applying M-Health to Palliative Care: A Systematic Review on the Use of M-Health in Monitoring Patients With Chronic Diseases and its Transposition in Palliative Care. *Am J Hosp Palliat Care*, 37, 549–564.

Brinkman-Stoppelenburg, A, Rietjens, JA, Van der Heide, A. 2014. The effects of advance care planning on end-of-life care: a systematic review. *Palliative medicine*, 28(8), 1000–1025.

Calton, B., Abedini, N. & Fratkin, M. 2020. Telemedicine in the Time of Coronavirus. *J Pain Symptom Manage*, 60, e12–e14.

Chakraborty, C., Pal, S., Bhattacharya, M., Dash, S. & Lee, S.-S. 2023. Overview of Chatbots with special emphasis on artificial intelligence-enabled ChatGPT in medical science. *Frontiers in artificial intelligence*, 6, 1237704.

Cook, D. J., Duncan, G., Sprint, G. & Fritz, R. L. 2018. Using smart city technology to make healthcare smarter. *Proceedings of the IEEE*, 106, 708–722.

Coughlan, S.,. 2025. *Kate reveals she is in remission from cancer* [Online]. bbc.co.uk. Available: https://www.bbc.co.uk/news/articles/cx2m8g2vp41o [Accessed 2nd April 2025].

Crosby, B., Hanchanale, S., Stanley, S. & Nwosu, A. C. 2021. Evaluating the use of video communication technology in a hospital specialist palliative care team during the COVID-19 pandemic. *AMRC Open Research*, 3, 5.

Dash, J., Haller, D. M., Sommer, J. & Junod Perron, N. 2016. Use of email, cell phone and text message between patients and primary-care physicians: cross-sectional study in a French-speaking part of Switzerland. *BMC health services research*, 16, 1–7.

Drago, W. A. & Wagner, R. J. 2004. Vark preferred learning styles and online education. *Management Research News*, 27, 1–13.

Engel, M., Kars, M. C., Teunissen, S. C. & van der Heide, A. 2023. Effective communication in palliative care from the perspectives of patients and relatives: a systematic review. *Palliative & supportive care*, 21, 890–913.

Fallowfield, L. J., Jenkins, V. A. & Beveridge, H. A. 2002. Truth may hurt but deceit hurts more: communication in palliative care. *Palliative medicine*, 16, 297–303.

Favela, J., Rodríguez, M., Preciado, A. & González, V. M. 2004. Integrating context-aware public displays into a mobile hospital information system. *IEEE transactions on information technology in Biomedicine*, 8, 279–286.

Fleming, N. D. 2001. *Teaching and learning styles: VARK strategies*, Neil Fleming.

Fridman, I., Johnson, S. & Elston Lafata, J. 2023. Health information and misinformation: A framework to guide research and Practice. *JMIR Medical Education*, 9, e38687.

Genovese, A., Borna, S., Gomez-Cabello, C. A., Haider, S. A., Prabha, S., Forte, A. J. & Veenstra, B. R. 2024. Artificial intelligence in clinical settings: a systematic review of its role in language translation and interpretation. *Annals of Translational Medicine*, 12, 117.

Greene, A., Greene, C. C. & Greene, C. 2019. Artificial intelligence, chatbots, and the future of medicine. *The Lancet Oncology*, 20, 481–482.

Hamidi, M., Mahendran, P. & Denecke, K. 2019. Towards a digital lean hospital: concept for a digital patient board and its integration with a hospital information system. *MEDINFO 2019: Health and Wellbeing e-Networks for All.* IOS Press.

Holt-Lunstad, J., Smith, T. B. & Layton, J. B. 2010. Social relationships and mortality risk: a meta-analytic review. *PLoS medicine*, 7, e1000316.

Ishizumi, A., Kolis, J., Abad, N., Prybylski, D., Brookmeyer, K. A., Voegeli, C., WARDLE, C. & CHIOU, H. 2024. Beyond misinformation: developing a public health prevention framework for managing information ecosystems. *The Lancet Public Health.*

Kate Granger. 2013. *#hello my name is…* [Online]. Available: https://www.hellomynameis.org.uk/ [Accessed 6th June 2024].

Kellehear, A. 2013. Compassionate communities: end-of-life care as everyone's responsibility. *QJM: An International Journal of Medicine*, 106, 1071–1075.

Kellehear, A. 2020. Compassionate cities: global significance and meaning for palliative care. *Progress in Palliative care*, 28, 115–119.

Kolb, D. A. 2007. *The Kolb learning style inventory*, Hay Resources Direct Boston, MA.

Kuwabara, A., Su, S. & Krauss, J. 2020. Utilizing digital health technologies for patient education in lifestyle medicine. *American journal of lifestyle medicine*, 14, 137–142.

MABEL AI. 2024. *Mabel Translate* [Online]. Available: https://mabel.care [Accessed].

Mackey, R. M., Yeow, M. E., Christensen, A. R., Ingram, C., Carey, E. C. & Lapid, M. I. 2020. Reconnecting: Strategies for Supporting Isolated Older Adults during COVID-19 through Tele-palliative Care. *Clinical gerontologist*, 1–8.

Matias, Y. & Leviathan, Y. 2018. Google Duplex: An AI System for Accomplish-ing Real-World Tasks Over the Phone.

National Institute for Research in Digital Science And Technology (INRIA), F.A.I.S.B.T.E.C.U.T.H.F.P.F.R.A.I.H.-I. 2024. Final Advisory Board recommendations—Socially Pertinent Robots in Gerontological Healthcare (SPRING).

Norris, J. & Taubert, M. 2020. How hospitals, hospices & other care facilities can use Video Calling apps, like Skype, to reduce isolation during the Coronavirus (COVID-19) pandemic. Available from: https://blogs.bmj.com/spcare/2020/03/15/using-skype-during-pandemic-isolation/ [Accessed 24th March 2025].

Nwosu, A. C., Monnery, D., Reid, V. L. & Chapman, L. 2017. Use of podcast technology to facilitate education, communication and dissemination in palliative care: the development of the AmiPal podcast. *BMJ Supportive & Palliative Care*, 7, 212–217.

O'Hara, J. K., Reynolds, C., Moore, S., Armitage, G., Sheard, L., Marsh, C., Watt, I., Wright, J. & Lawton, R. 2018. What can patients tell us about the quality and safety of hospital care? Findings from a UK multicentre survey study. *BMJ quality & safety*, 27, 673–682.

Popowicz, D. M. 2021. "Doctor Knows Best": On the Epistemic Authority of the Medical Practitioner. *Philosophy of Medicine*, 2.

Pruchno, R. 2019. Technology and aging: An evolving partnership. Oxford University Press US.

Rao, P., Mcgee, L. M. & Seideman, C. A. 2024. A Comparative assessment of ChatGPT vs. Google Translate for the translation of patient instructions. *Journal of Medical Artificial Intelligence*, 7.

Raza, M. A., Aziz, S., Noreen, M., Saeed, A., Anjum, I., Ahmed, M. & Raza, S. M. 2022. Artificial intelligence (AI) in pharmacy: an overview of innovations. *INNOVATIONS in pharmacy*, 13, https://doi.org/10.24926/iip.v13i2.4839.

Sam Haysom. 2022. *The queue to see the Queen is miles long. It has its own YouTube livestream* [Online]. Mashable. Available: https://mashable.com/article/queue-tracker-livestream-queen-lying-in-state-what3words [Accessed 4th June 20244].

Sandhu, S. K., Kouvroukoglou, N., Campodonico, M. & Mehendale, F. 2022. Lost in translation: a caution against using automated and commercial translation services for medical communications. *BMJ Global Health*, 7, e008067.

Stanley, S., Finucane, A., Thompson, A. & Nwosu, A. C. 2024. How can technology be used to support communication in palliative care beyond the covid-19 pandemic: a mixed-methods national survey of palliative care healthcare professionals. *BMC palliative care*, 23, 40.

Taubert, M., Watts, G., Boland, J. & Radbruch, L. 2014. Palliative social media. *BMJ Supportive & Palliative Care*, 4, 13–18.

The Academy of Medical Sciences 2018. Our data-driven future in healthcare. Website of the Academy of Medical Sciences.

Timmers, T., Janssen, L., Kool, R. B. & Kremer, J. A. 2020. Educating patients by providing timely information using smartphone and tablet apps: systematic review. *Journal of medical Internet research*, 22, e17342.

Toplo, E. 2019. Preparing the healthcare workforce to deliver the digital future the Topol Review: an Independent Report on Behalf of the Secretary of State for Health and Social Care. NHS Health Education, London, UK.

Zawati, M. N. H. & Lang, M. 2024. Does an app a day keep the doctor away? AI symptom checker applications, entrenched bias, and professional responsibility. *Journal of Medical Internet Research*, 26, e50344.

5 Older People, Long-Term Conditions and the Potential for New Technologies

5.1 The Challenge

Many countries are required to address the challenge to provide the appropriate infrastructure to manage the needs of aging populations. The number of people aged 65 years or older worldwide is projected to increase by greater than double, rising from 761 million in 2021 to 1.6 billion in 2050 (United Nations: Department of Economic and Social Affairs, 2023). The number of people aged 80 years or older is growing even faster. As people live longer, they are more likely to develop diseases associated with aging. Commonly, this includes conditions like cancer but also includes other long-term conditions (describing physical health conditions that require ongoing management over a period of years). Examples of long-term conditions include diabetes mellitus, chronic obstructive pulmonary disease (COPD) (and other respiratory problems), obesity, heart problems and dementia (World Health Organization, 2024). There is potential to explore opportunities to use technologies to create innovative solutions to provide care, and support people to self-manage their health.

5.2 What's in This Chapter?

This chapter outlines the practical considerations associated with long-term conditions in older people and discusses some opportunities to use technologies to provide support for people, and their caregivers. Specifically, this chapter outlines the opportunities to use technology to support the evolving needs of an older person living with a long-term medical condition. The focus of this chapter is on a person who is living in their own environment, who is trying to remain independent by using AgeTech solutions to support their physical function. We use the persona of Khalid to describe some of the practical

A. C. Nwosu et al., *Technologies in Palliative Care for Older People*, Synthesis Lectures on Technology and Health, https://doi.org/10.1007/978-3-032-04277-4_5

opportunities of using technologies to support his palliative care needs, which have been caused by his diagnosis of Parkinson's disease. Kahlid's story demonstrates the potential to use AgeTech solutions to manage his care needs. We hope the themes covered in this chapter are transferable to other people with different illnesses who are affected by similar problems. The chapter concludes with examples of some promising digital interventions.

5.3 Persona and Scenario—Khalid

Persona: Khalid (86), a resilient elderly gentleman, faces the daily challenges of Parkinson's disease (a progressive neurological disorder that primarily affects movement, causing symptoms like tremors, slowness of movement, and stiffness, due to a loss of brain cells that produce dopamine (Dauer and Przedborski, 2003)) with curiosity in embracing technological advancements. Khalid's journey with Parkinson's disease has been positively influenced by various technologies designed to enhance his quality-of-life (Fig. 5.1).

Scenario: Khalid embodies resilience and determination as he faces the daily challenges of Parkinson's disease. He lives in Paris, which is far from his family. Khalid relies on

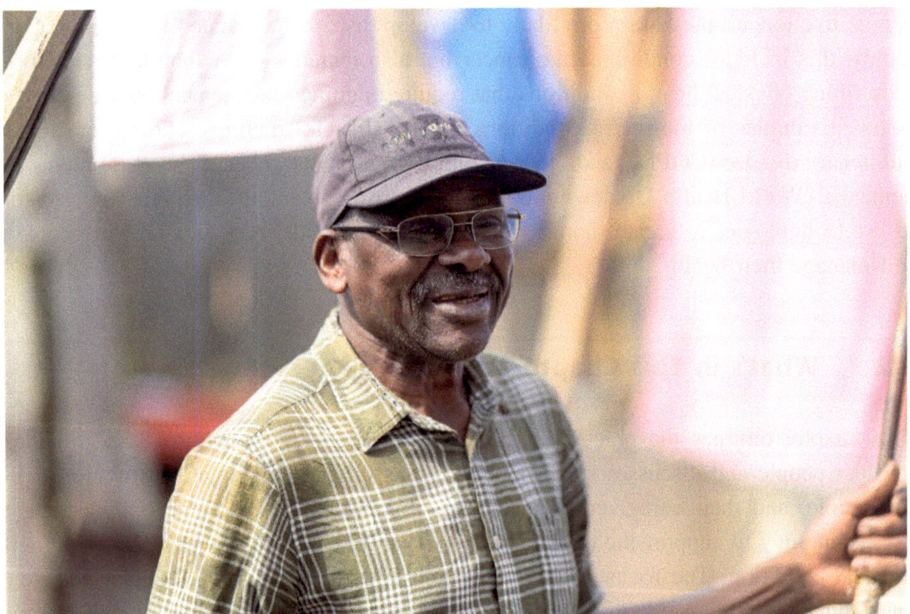

Fig. 5.1 *Credit* David Tett/aging better

the support of his neighbors and embraces technology to aid his mobility and maintain his independence. Despite his condition, Khalid refuses to let Parkinson's disease define him. With the help of his supportive neighbors, who often check in on him and assist with tasks when needed, he manages to navigate through his daily routine with dignity.

Solution: Technology plays a crucial role in Khalid's life, allowing him to overcome many obstacles. He uses assistive devices such as a walker, with advanced stability features, and a smartphone equipped with voice recognition software. With the smartphone, he can make calls, send messages, and control his home appliances with voice commands, making tasks more manageable. Additionally, Khalid uses wearable devices that track his movements and provide feedback on his balance and gait. These devices help him monitor his condition and adjust his activities, minimizing the risk of falls and injuries. Moreover, Khalid stays connected with his family through video calls, allowing him to share moments and updates with them despite the distance. He finds comfort and joy in these interactions, knowing that (even though they are physically apart) his family is still there for him. Khalid uses the following technologies to help maintain his independence and continues to lead a fulfilling life despite the challenges of Parkinson's disease.

Telemedicine and Virtual Consultations: Khalid has found telemedicine helpful, a platform that allows him to consult with his neurology team from the comfort of his own home. This has been especially beneficial on days when his mobility is limited, sparing him the arduous 26-mile journey to the clinic. Through virtual consultations, Khalid can discuss his symptoms, medication adjustments, and receive professional advice on managing his condition effectively.

Wearable Devices and Fitness Trackers: Khalid's wearable device has become a faithful companion. It monitors his movement patterns, sleep quality, and heart rate, providing valuable insights into his overall health. Khalid uses the data from his wearables to make informed decisions about his daily activities, ensuring he balances his energy between rest and physical exertion. And he also sets himself targets; for example, his daily step-count.

Deep Brain Stimulation* via *implanted brain electrodes: Khalid had a Deep Brain Stimulation (DBS) device inserted, beacause his medication treatment had become less effective over the past 7 years. DBS is a neurosurgical procedure that uses implanted electrodes and electrical stimulation to treat movement disorders associated with Parkinson's disease (PD), essential tremor, dystonia and other neurological conditions (Benabid, 2003). The electrodes are connected to an implanted pulse generator which is battery powered. DBS improves symptoms by delivering electrical impulses directly to targeted areas deep within the brain, overriding abnormal brain-cell firing patterns arising in Parkinson's disease.

Successful DBS allows a decrease in medication or makes a medication regimen more tolerable. There are gains in movement and control. The intervention is used for carefully selected patients, in accordance with clinical eligibility criteria, who cannot be adequately controlled with drugs or whose drugs have severe side effects. Khalid has been able to discontinue some of his medication and reduce others, due to this procedure. Newer DBS devices are being trialed, including some that are much smaller than Khalid's, which may help shorten and simplify the procedure to implant a DBS device, reducing time in theatre, complexity, the cost, and hopefully increasing reported levels of patient satisfaction. It may also reduce the need for patients requiring further surgery to repair damaged wires (BBC News, 2022).

Medication Management Apps: Khalid uses a medication management app to help him manage his complex medication regimen (Morawski et al., 2018). The app provides Khalid with timely reminders and dosage tracking, which means he no longer struggles to remember if he has taken his medications. Furthermore, Khalid has connected his medication management app to his smart speaker (a speaker that connects to the internet and can be controlled by voice commands (Bienfait et al., 2020). The virtual assistant on the smart speaker uses voice prompts to remind Khalid to take his medications (Basile et al., 2024). The medication app has improved Khalid's confidence in taking his medications, which has improved his overall well-being.

Virtual Reality for Pain Management: Khalid uses VR to treat chronic pain during his weekly visits to the neurology rehabilitation center. Khalid enjoys the immersive VR experiences, which provides distraction from his symptoms and the creates opportunity for him to encounter new experiences (Mo et al., 2022, Martin et al., 2022). Because of this positive experience, Khalid bought his own VR kit to use at home. At home he uses VR to walk on a beach and trek through a forest. This innovative approach to pain management has become an invaluable tool in Khalid's daily routine.

Smart Home Technology: Khalid's living space has been transformed by smart home technology (Liu et al., 2016). Voice-activated controls for lights, thermostats, and security systems have given Khalid greater sense of control, especially when he is unable to move his hands and arms, and he finds it hard to operate the lights in his home. Khalid uses technology to navigate around his home, using the tools to control his environment in ways previously unimaginable. Khalid's daughter has set up the washing machine so that he can easily program it either from his computer, or via voice activation.

5.4 How Older People Experience Decline in Their Physical Health and Symptoms

Khalid's story illustrates the physical health problems associated with aging. As people age, they typically experience a natural decline in their physical health due to a combination of genetic factors, lifestyle choices, and environmental influences (World Health Organization, 2024). Based on Khalid's example, it is important that AgeTech interventions are designed to meet the changing physiological requirements of people as they age. The aging process can vary significantly from person to person, but there are some common trends and symptoms associated with aging. These are outlined below:

Muscle Mass and Strength: Muscle mass and strength decrease as people age; this is known as sarcopenia. Sarcopenia often starts when people reach their 30 s or 40 s but it becomes more pronounced after the age of 50. As muscle mass decreases, it can lead to reduced mobility and instability (Volpi et al., 2004).

Bone Density: Older individuals tend to experience a decrease in bone density, which can lead to conditions like osteoporosis. This makes bones more fragile and prone to fractures (Smit et al., 2024).

Joint Health: The joints may become stiffer and less flexible due to a reduction in the production of synovial fluid, which lubricates the joints. Conditions like arthritis can become more common, causing pain, swelling, and reduced mobility (Sacitharan, 2019).

Cardiovascular System: The cardiovascular system undergoes changes, as arteries may become less flexible and narrower, leading to higher blood pressure. This can increase the risk of heart disease and other cardiovascular conditions (Lye and Donnellan, 2000).

Respiratory Function: Lung capacity tends to decrease with age, which can result in reduced stamina and endurance. This may result in increased fatigue during physical activities (Janssens et al., 1999).

Vision and Hearing: Changes in vision, such as presbyopia (difficulty focusing on close objects) and cataracts, become more common. Hearing loss is also a common age-related issue (Owsley, 2011).

Metabolism: The metabolic rate tends to decrease, which can lead to weight gain if dietary habits remain the same. This is partly due to a decrease in muscle mass and activity level (Costantino et al., 2016).

Digestive System: The digestive system may become less efficient, leading to issues like constipation or difficulty absorbing certain nutrients. This can be exacerbated by changes in diet and reduced physical activity (Soenen et al., 2016).

Skin Changes: The skin becomes thinner, less elastic, and more prone to wrinkles. It also becomes more susceptible to bruises and injuries (Baumann, 2007).

Cognitive Function: While not strictly a physical symptom, cognitive decline is a common concern in older age. This can manifest as difficulty with memory, processing speed, and multitasking. In some cases, it can lead to conditions like dementia or Alzheimer's disease (Christensen, 2001).

Immune System: Aging is associated with a number of changes in the immune system, meaning that the immune responses of older people are less effective, making older individuals more susceptible to infections and illnesses (Effros, 2001).

Pain and Discomfort: Chronic pain, often associated with conditions like arthritis, becomes more prevalent with age. This can impact mobility and overall quality-of-life (Abdulla et al., 2013).

Although these factors are typical of aging, they are not uniform across all individuals. Lifestyle choices, genetics, and overall health can significantly influence the aging process. Healthy aging can be promoted through lifestyle factors such as regular exercise, good nutrition, and appropriate medical care (Beard et al., 2016). Therefore, there is potential that AgeTech can be used to improve physical function, psychosocial health and quality-of-life by modifying aspects associated with aging (Sixsmith and Cosco, 2024, Sixsmith, 2021).

5.5 How Technology Can Be Used to Improve Palliative Care for Older People with Long-Term Conditions

Using Khalid's story, there are potential opportunities to use AgeTech to support palliative care. Examples include the following.

Telehealth and Remote Monitoring: Telehealth allows older adults to consult with healthcare providers from the comfort of their homes (Bonsignore et al., 2018). Video consultations can facilitate discussions about treatment options, adjustments in medications, and lifestyle recommendations. Remote monitoring devices can track vital signs, medication adherence, and other health metrics, providing timely feedback and alerts to healthcare providers (Hancock et al., 2019). For example, Personal Emergency Response Systems (PERS), also known as telecare or personal alarms, are electronic devices that alert call centers or carers if someone experiences a problem, like a fall, and needs assistance. They often include wearable devices with a button that, when pressed, connects the user to a trained operator who can send help (Stokke, 2016) (Fig. 5.2).

Wearables These technologies have been used to provide a range of monitoring functions for users, such as recording physical activity, heart rate, sleep patterns, and other health metrics (Pavic et al., 2020). Wearables can track vital signs, pain levels, and other relevant metrics, sending this information to healthcare providers, which allows for early intervention and adjustment of treatment plans (Nwosu et al., 2018; Haghi et al., 2017). Smart Clothing (garments that incorporate technology, like sensors and electronics, to monitor body data, adapt to the environment, or perform specific functions) is a growing area in wearable technology, with some clothing featuring embedded technologies (e.g. heat or cold therapy) to alleviate pain and discomfort (Axisa et al., 2005).

Assistive technologies and Robotics: Technologies like walkers, canes, and wheelchairs are designed to enhance mobility and independence for individuals with mobility issues. Assistive devices encompass all types of physical assistance aids, whilst mobility devices specifically describe aids related to physical movement (Yusif et al., 2016). Assistive

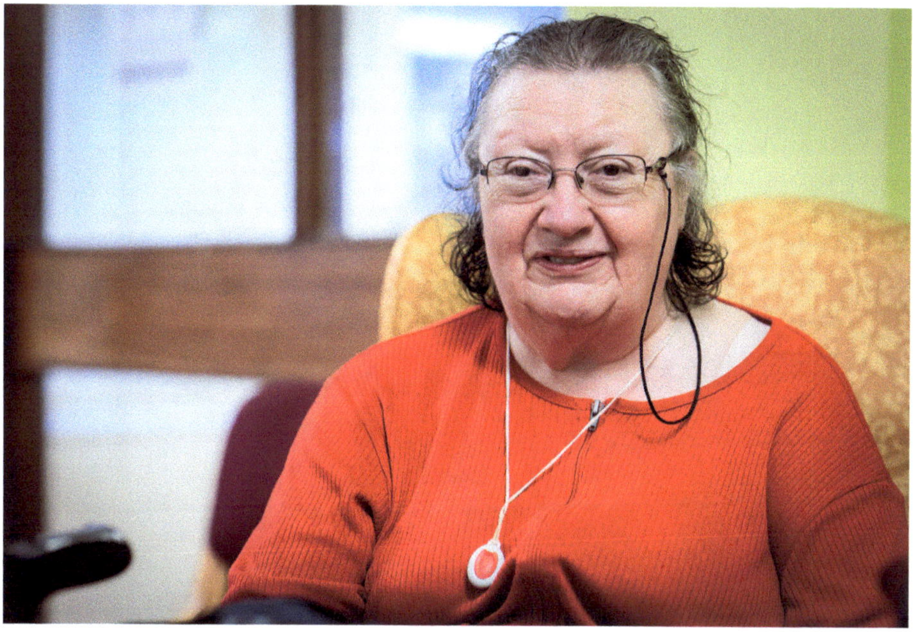

Fig. 5.2 An example of a personal emergency response systems alarm button, which alerts a trained operator to send help to the individual who presses the button. Connected home and Internet of Things (IoT) devices, personal emergency response alarms and other such devices are now internet-enabled, facilitating connection (and transmission of data) with healthcare providers. *Credit* Aging Better

technology also includes advanced exoskeletons and robotic exosuits (Grimmer et al., 2019). A robotic exoskeleton is a mechanical device worn by a human being for certain purposes or applications, with the potential to augment human strength (Kong and Jeon, 2006). Comparatively, an exosuit is a soft wearable robot that uses innovative textiles to provide a more conformal, unobtrusive and compliant means to interface with the human body. Exosuits augment the capabilities of people (e.g., improved walking efficiency) and can improve mobility and function for people with muscle weakness, physical and neurological disorders (Awad et al., 2017) (Figs. 5.3 and 5.4).

Robots are being developed to assist with daily tasks such as cleaning, cooking, and the provision of companionship for older individuals (Nwosu et al., 2019b). Robots can assist with mobility for those with mobility issues or chronic pain, providing support for walking (Bemelmans et al., 2012). For example, the SPRING (Socially Assistive Robots in Gerontological healthcare) trial developed robots equipped with advanced artificial intelligence to enable natural conversations, understand patient needs, and assist hospital staff with routine tasks in experiments with elderly volunteers (National Institute for Research in Digital Science and Technology (INRIA), 2024).

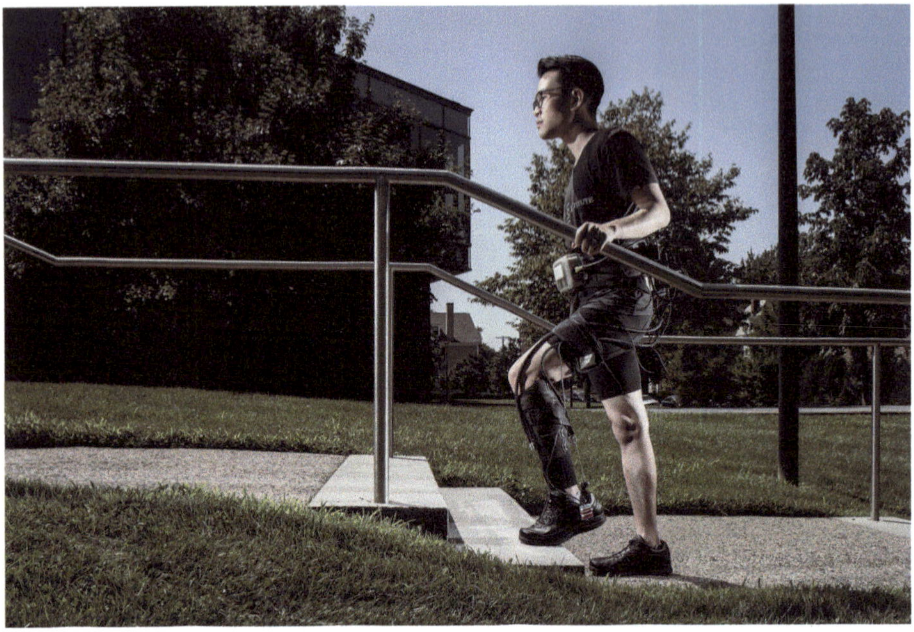

Fig. 5.3 Examples of a soft robotics system developed by Harvard Biodesign lab. *Credit* Harvard Biodesign lab

Box 5.1

Next-generation socially assistive robots have been successfully tested in a healthcare setting to assist patients, alleviate their anxiety, and relieve pressure on nursing staff as part of a hospital trial co-conducted by researchers from the National Robotarium in Paris, France. The SPRING (Socially Assistive Robots in Gerontological healthcare) trial developed robots equipped with advanced artificial intelligence to enable natural conversations, understand patient needs, and assist hospital staff with routine tasks across three waves of experiments with elderly volunteers at Assistance Publique Hôpitaux de Paris. Results show that robots were able to smoothly engage in social interactions like greeting patients, answering questions, and providing directions. Critically, robots are quickly demonstrating an ability to comprehend multi-party conversations—following dialogue between several individuals simultaneously (National Institute for Research in Digital Science and Technology - INRIA, 2024).

Smart homes and sensor-based Monitoring: Devices like smart thermostats, lighting, and security systems can be controlled via voice commands or mobile apps, making

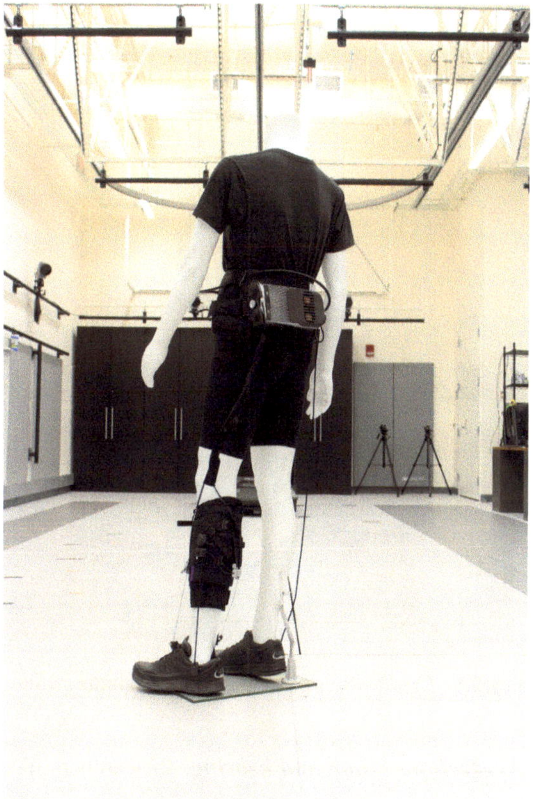

Fig. 5.4 Examples of a soft robotics system developed by Harvard Biodesign lab. *Credit* Harvard Biodesign lab

it easier for older adults to manage their living spaces and maintain independence (Liu et al., 2016). Technologies like motion sensors and wearable devices can detect changes in movement patterns, alerting caregivers or healthcare providers if a fall or unusual activity is detected. Smart mattresses, sleep tracking devices and neurostimulation tools can be used to monitor and improve sleep quality (Future Today Strategy Group, 2025) (Fig. 5.5).

Virtual Reality (VR) and Augmented Reality (AR): VR can be used to manage physical therapy, pain management, and cognitive training (Martin et al., 2022; Mo et al., 2022). VR can be used to distract individuals from pain, reducing their perception of discomfort. VR has been used effectively for procedures, physical therapy, and chronic pain management (Martin et al., 2022). AR, in combination with conventional therapy, has been used for the treatment of balance and fall prevention in geriatrics, lower and upper limb functionality in stroke, phantom pain syndrome, and to improve walking ability in people with Parkinson's disease (Gil et al., 2021).

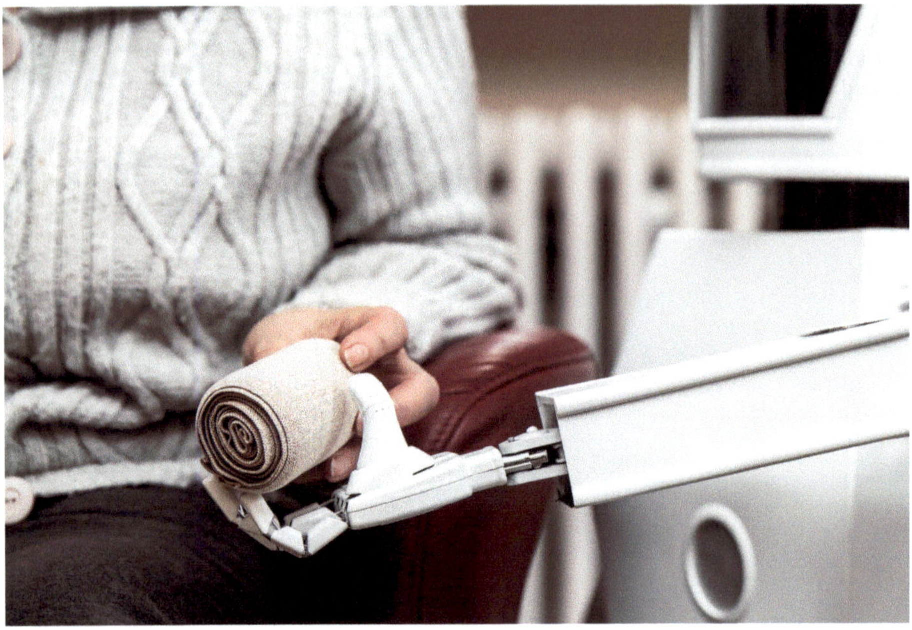

Fig. 5.5 *Credit* Miriam Doerr Martin Frommherz/Shutterstock

AgeTech for vision and hearing: Researchers have proposed that smart glasses (eyewear that integrates technology, often including cameras, displays, audio, and Bluetooth connectivity, allowing users to access information, interact with digital content, and perform various tasks hands-free) can empower patients by increasing opportunities to interact with healthcare providers, family and other patients (Wrzesińska, 2015). Innovations in hearing technology offer opportunities to support older adults with hearing loss. For example, hearing test assessments (traditionally only available in a clinical setting) can now be done at home with smartphone-based applications (Irace et al., 2021) and smart home speakers (Ooster et al., 2020). Researchers have highlighted potential developments of assistive technology for hearing, including innovations in hearing aids, implant devices and the need for website developers to make content more accessible for hearing-impaired users, by developing technology which translates web-based speech and text into various sign languages (Hermawati and Pieri, 2020).

Mobile devices and applications (Apps): Mobile devices (such as smartphones and tablets) and apps can provide users with greater control to manage their health (Bienfait et al., 2020). Examples may include Cognitive Fitness apps, which provide brain-training exercises to improve cognitive function and memory retention. Nutrition and diet apps to help users track their dietary intake, offer healthy recipes, and provide nutritional advice tailored to the user's needs (Almasri et al., 2024). Symptom management apps to help users directly report problems (such as pain), and log information about their health status, experiences, and quality-of-life (i.e. electronic patient outcome measures—ePROMs) (Benze et al., 2019), which can be shared with healthcare providers to inform treatment decisions. Medication management apps can provide reminders for medication schedules, track dosages, and send alerts to caregivers or healthcare providers if doses are missed (Tabi et al., 2019). Some medication apps may facilitate prescription refills, by sending messages to the user's pharmacy or healthcare professional. Biofeedback and Relaxation Apps can teach users techniques, like deep breathing, progressive muscle relaxation, and guided imagery to help individuals manage pain and reduce stress (Mikolasek et al., 2021).

Pain and symptom management technologies: AgeTech devices can support assessment and management of palliative conditions in older people. Examples include, the evaluation and management of pain with transcutaneous electrical nerve stimulation (TENS) units, ultrasound therapy, AR and VR (Waqar et al., 2017). There is growing evidence about the use of non-invasive technologies in the management of problems experienced by older people. For example, Bispectral Index (BIS) monitoring (which uses electroencephalographic data to assess consciousness levels), has been used to titrate medications doses in people who lack the ability to adequately describe their symptoms (e.g. people who lack capacity due to conditions such as dementia) (Monreal-Carrillo et al., 2017, Barbato, 2001). Bioelectrical impedance analysis (a non-invasive technology to assess body composition) has been used to measure body composition and hydration in older people with advanced cancer (Nwosu et al., 2019a, 2016). Also, non-invasive technologies have been used to treat insomnia, by using non-invasive brain stimulation to promote, and enhance sleep quality (Bressler et al., 2024; Fehér et al., 2021).

Online Resources: Many online resources are available to provide support and advice for people, for numerous medical problems. Social media, blogging, YouTube and others create opportunities for patients to access information and take ownership of their health (Taubert et al., 2014; Easwar et al., 2022). Furthermore, online resources have been developed by healthcare providers to help the public find information about available healthcare services. For example, in the UK the National Health Service (NHS) provides a website (https://www.nhs.uk) and app to help citizens to coordinate their healthcare. Implementing these technologies requires consideration of individual needs, preferences, and levels of technological literacy. It is important to ensure that these technologies are accessible, trustworthy, user-friendly, and address the needs of older adults (Sixsmith, 2021).

5.6 Artificial Intelligence Applications in Palliative Care for Long-Term Conditions

Artificial Intelligence is being used by practitioners for pain and symptom management in long-term conditions, such as dementia. For example, PainChek (PainChek Ltd, Sydney, Australia—https://www.painchek.com/uk/) is a smart-device system application, which combines AI facial recognition technology and smart automation with digital pain checklists (Brett and Severn, 2023). Caregivers can use the PainChek system to assist pain assessments (especially in people with communication difficulties who may struggle to describe their pain), which can help care providers to deliver pain management plans (Pu et al., 2023).

5.7 Key Initiatives

The European Innovation Partnership on Active and Healthy Aging (EIP on AHA).

The European Innovation Partnership in Active and Healthy Aging (AHA) is an initiative that aims to foster innovative use of digital health for active and healthy aging. The European Innovation Partnership (an EIP) aims to strengthen the European Union (EU) research and innovation, by bringing together relevant actors at EU, national and regional levels across different policy areas to address a specific societal challenge. The EIP on AHA was the first EIP created in 2011. It focuses on demographic change and the active and healthy aging of the people of Europe.

https://digital-strategy.ec.europa.eu/en/policies/eip-aha.

Assistive Technology 2030: Life Changing Assistive Technology for All Global disability innovation hub.

The UK Aid-funded AT2030 program tests what works to improve access to life-changing Assistive Technology (AT) for all. This project is operating in over 40 countries in partnership with over 70 global delivery partners, https://at2030.org/at/.

5.8 Find Out More

Socially Pertinent Robots in Gerontological Healthcare—SPRING.

https://spring-h2020.eu/.

Harvard Biodesign Lab.

https://biodesign.seas.harvard.edu/soft-exosuits.

https://www.technologyreview.com/2023/01/09/1065135/japan-automating-eldercare-robots/.

References

Abdulla, A., Adams, N., Bone, M., Elliott, A. M., Gaffin, J., Jones, D., Knaggs, R., Martin, D., Sampson, L. & Schofield, P. 2013. Guidance on the management of pain in older people. *Age and ageing*, 42, i1–57.

Almasri, A., El-Kour, T. Y., Silva, L. & Abdulfattah, Y. 2024. Evaluating the Energy Efficiency of Popular US Smartphone Health Care Apps: Comparative Analysis Study Toward Sustainable Health and Nutrition Apps Practices. *JMIR Human Factors*, 11, e58311.

Awad, L. N., Bae, J., O'Donnell, K., de Rossi, S. M., Hendron, K., Sloot, L. H., Kudzia, P., Allen, S., Holt, K. G. & Ellis, T. D. 2017. A soft robotic exosuit improves walking in patients after stroke. *Science translational medicine*, 9, eaai9084.

Axisa, F., Schmitt, P. M., Gehin, C., Delhomme, G., Mcadams, E. & Dittmar, A. 2005. Flexible technologies and smart clothing for citizen medicine, home healthcare, and disease prevention. *IEEE Transactions on information technology in biomedicine*, 9, 325–336.

Barbato, M. 2001. Bispectral index monitoring in unconscious palliative care patients. *Journal of Palliative Care*, 17, 102–108.

Basile, I., Consolo, L., Colombo, S., Rusconi, D., Rampichini, F. & Lusignani, M. 2024. Technology to support older adults in home palliative care: a scoping review. *American Journal of Hospice and Palliative Medicine®*, 41, 673–690.

Baumann, L. 2007. Skin ageing and its treatment. *The Journal of Pathology: A Journal of the Pathological Society of Great Britain and Ireland*, 211, 241–251.

BBC NEWS. 2022. *Parkinson's disease symptoms 'reversed' by mini implant, trial suggests* [Online]. Available: https://www.bbc.co.uk/news/uk-england-bristol-61215241 [Accessed 24th March 2025].

Beard, J. R., Officer, A., de Carvalho, I. A., Sadana, R., Pot, A. M., Michel, J.-P., Lloyd-Sherlock, P., Epping-Jordan, J. E., Peeters, G. G. & Mahanani, W. R. 2016. The World report on ageing and health: a policy framework for healthy ageing. *The lancet*, 387, 2145–2154.

Bemelmans, R., Gelderblom, G. J., Jonker, P. & de Witte, L. 2012. Socially assistive robots in elderly care: a systematic review into effects and effectiveness. *Journal of the American Medical Directors Association*, 13, 114–120. e1.

Benabid, A. L. 2003. Deep brain stimulation for Parkinson's disease. *Current opinion in neurobiology*, 13, 696–706.

Benze, G., Nauck, F., Alt-Epping, B., Gianni, G., Bauknecht, T., Ettl, J., Munte, A., Kretzschmar, L. & Gaertner, J. 2019. PROutine: a feasibility study assessing surveillance of electronic patient reported outcomes and adherence via smartphone app in advanced cancer. *Ann Palliat Med*, 8, 104–111.

Bienfait, F., Petit, M., Pardenaud, R., Guineberteau, C. & Pignon, A. 2020. Applying M-Health to Palliative Care: A Systematic Review on the Use of M-Health in Monitoring Patients With Chronic Diseases and its Transposition in Palliative Care. *Am J Hosp Palliat Care*, 37, 549–564.

Bonsignore, L., Bloom, N., Steinhauser, K., Nichols, R., Allen, T., Twaddle, M. & Bull, J. 2018. Evaluating the feasibility and acceptability of a telehealth program in a rural palliative care population: TapCloud for palliative care. *Journal of pain and symptom management*, 56, 7–14.

Bressler, S., Neely, R., Yost, R. M. & Wang, D. 2024. A randomized controlled trial of alpha phase-locked auditory stimulation to treat symptoms of sleep onset insomnia. *Scientific reports*, 14, 13039.

Brett, K. & Severn, M. 2023. Facial analysis technology for pain detection: a potentially useful tool for people living with dementia. *Canadian Journal of Health Technologies*, 3.

Christensen, H. 2001. What cognitive changes can be expected with normal ageing? *Australian & New Zealand Journal of Psychiatry*, 35, 768–775.

Costantino, S., Paneni, F. & Cosentino, F. 2016. Ageing, metabolism and cardiovascular disease. *The Journal of physiology*, 594, 2061–2073.

Dauer, W. & Przedborski, S. 2003. Parkinson's disease: mechanisms and models. *Neuron*, 39, 889–909.

Easwar, S., Alonzi, S., Hirsch, J., Mossman, B. & Hoerger, M. 2022. Palliative Care TikTok: Describing the Landscape and Explaining Social Media Engagement. *Journal of Palliative Medicine*, 26, 360–365.

Effros, R. B. Ageing and the immune system. Ageing Vulnerability: Causes and Interventions: Novartis Foundation Symposium 235, 2001. Wiley Online Library, 130–145.

Fehér, K. D., Wunderlin, M., Maier, J. G., Hertenstein, E., Schneider, C. L., Mikutta, C., Züst, M. A., Klöppel, S. & Nissen, C. 2021. Shaping the slow waves of sleep: A systematic and integrative review of sleep slow wave modulation in humans using non-invasive brain stimulation. *Sleep medicine reviews*, 58, 101438.

Future Today Strategy Group 2025. 2025 Tech Trend Report.

Gil, M. J. V., Gonzalez-Medina, G., Lucena-Anton, D., Perez-Cabezas, V., Ruiz-Molinero, M. D. C. & Martín-Valero, R. 2021. Augmented reality in physical therapy: systematic review and meta-analysis. *JMIR Serious Games*, 9, e30985.

Grimmer, M., Riener, R., Walsh, C. J. & Seyfarth, A. 2019. Mobility related physical and functional losses due to aging and disease-a motivation for lower limb exoskeletons. *Journal of neuroengineering and rehabilitation*, 16, 1–21.

Haghi, M., Thurow, K. & Stoll, R. 2017. Wearable Devices in Medical Internet of Things: Scientific Research and Commercially Available Devices. *Healthc Inform Res*, 23, 4–15.

Hancock, S., Preston, N., Jones, H. & Gadoud, A. 2019. Telehealth in palliative care is being described but not evaluated: a systematic review. *BMC Palliative Care*, 18, 114.

Hermawati, S. & Pieri, K. 2020. Assistive technologies for severe and profound hearing loss: Beyond hearing aids and implants. *Assistive Technology.*

Irace, A. L., Sharma, R. K., Reed, N. S. & Golub, J. S. 2021. Smartphone-based applications to detect hearing loss: a review of current technology. *Journal of the American Geriatrics Society*, 69, 307–316.

Janssens, J.-P., Pache, J.-C. & Nicod, L. 1999. Physiological changes in respiratory function associated with ageing. *European Respiratory Journal*, 13, 197–205.

Kong, K. & Jeon, D. 2006. Design and control of an exoskeleton for the elderly and patients. *IEEE/ASME Transactions on mechatronics*, 11, 428–432.

Liu, L., Stroulia, E., Nikolaidis, I., Miguel-Cruz, A. & Rios Rincon, A. 2016. Smart homes and home health monitoring technologies for older adults: A systematic review. *Int J Med Inform*, 91, 44–59.

Lye, M. & Donnellan, C. 2000. Heart disease in the elderly. *Heart*, 84, 560–566.

Martin, J. L., Saredakis, D., Hutchinson, A. D., Crawford, G. B. & Loetscher, T. 2022. Virtual Reality in Palliative Care: A Systematic Review. *Healthcare (Basel)*, 10.

Mikolasek, M., Witt, C. M. & Barth, J. 2021. Effects and implementation of a mindfulness and relaxation app for patients with cancer: Mixed methods feasibility study. *JMIR cancer*, 7, e16785.

Mo, J., Vickerstaff, V., Minton, O., Tavabie, S., Taubert, M., Stone, P. & White, N. 2022. How effective is virtual reality technology in palliative care? A systematic review and meta-analysis. *Palliat Med*, 36, 1047–1058.

Monreal-Carrillo, E., Allende-Pérez, S., Hui, D., García-Salamanca, M.-F., Bruera, E. & Verástegui, E. 2017. Bispectral Index monitoring in cancer patients undergoing palliative sedation: a preliminary report. *Supportive Care in Cancer*, 25, 3143–3149.

Morawski, K., Ghazinouri, R., Krumme, A., Lauffenburger, J. C., Lu, Z., Durfee, E., Oley, L., Lee, J., Mohta, N. & Haff, N. 2018. Association of a smartphone application with medication adherence and blood pressure control: the MedISAFE-BP randomized clinical trial. *JAMA internal medicine*, 178, 802–809.

National Institute for Research in Digital Science And Technology (INRIA), F.A.I.S.B.T.E.C.U.T.H.F.P.F.R.A.I.H.-I. 2024. Final Advisory Board recommendations—Socially Pertinent Robots in Gerontological Healthcare (SPRING).

Nwosu, A. C., Mayland, C. R., Mason, S., Cox, T. F., Varro, A. & Ellershaw, J. 2016. The association of hydration status with physical signs, symptoms and survival in advanced cancer—The use of bioelectrical impedance vector analysis (BIVA) technology to evaluate fluid volume in palliative care: An observational study. *PLoS One*, 11, e0163114.

Nwosu, A. C., Quinn, C., Samuels, J., Mason, S. & Payne, T. R. 2018. Wearable smartwatch technology to monitor symptoms in advanced illness. *BMJ supportive & palliative care*, 8, 237–237.

Nwosu, A. C., Mayland, C. R., Mason, S., Cox, T. F., Varro, A., Stanley, S. & Ellershaw, J. 2019a. Bioelectrical impedance vector analysis (BIVA) as a method to compare body composition differences according to cancer stage and type. *Clinical nutrition ESPEN*, 30, 59–66.

Nwosu, A. C., Sturgeon, B., Mcglinchey, T., Goodwin, C. D., Behera, A., Mason, S., Stanley, S. & PAYNE, T. R. 2019b. Robotic technology for palliative and supportive care: Strengths, weaknesses, opportunities and threats. *Palliat Med*, 33, 1106–1113.

Ooster, J., Krueger, M., Bach, J.-H., Wagener, K. C., Kollmeier, B. & Meyer, B. T. 2020. Speech audiometry at home: Automated listening tests via smart speakers with normal-hearing and hearing-impaired listeners. *Trends in Hearing*, 24, 2331216520970011.

Owsley, C. 2011. Aging and vision. *Vision research*, 51, 1610–1622.

Pavic, M., Klaas, V., Theile, G., Kraft, J., Tröster, G. & Guckenberger, M. 2020. Feasibility and Usability Aspects of Continuous Remote Monitoring of Health Status in Palliative Cancer Patients Using Wearables. *Oncology*, 98, 386–395.

Pu, L., Coppieters, M. W., Smalbrugge, M., Jones, C., Byrnes, J., Todorovic, M. & Moyle, W. 2023. Implementing PainChek and PARO to support pain assessment and management in residents with dementia: a qualitative study. *Pain Management Nursing*, 24, 587–594.

Sacitharan, P. K. 2019. Ageing and osteoarthritis. *Biochemistry and cell biology of ageing: part II clinical science*, 123–159.

Sixsmith, A. & Cosco, T. 2024. Technology, aging, and mental health: opportunities and challenges. *Aging & Mental Health*, 28, i–iii.

Sixsmith, A. 2021. AgeTech: Technology-based solutions for aging societies. *Promoting the health of older adults: the Canadian experience*, 135.

Smit, A., Meijer, O. & Winter, E. 2024. The multi-faceted nature of age-associated osteoporosis. *Bone Reports*, 101750.

Soenen, S., Rayner, C. K., Jones, K. L. & Horowitz, M. 2016. The ageing gastrointestinal tract. *Current Opinion in Clinical Nutrition & Metabolic Care*, 19, 12–18.

Stokke, R. 2016. The personal emergency response system as a technology innovation in primary health care services: an integrative review. *Journal of medical Internet research*, 18, e187.

Tabi, K., Randhawa, A. S., Choi, F., Mithani, Z., Albers, F., Schnieder, M., Nikoo, M., Vigo, D., Jang, K. & Demlova, R. 2019. Mobile apps for medication management: review and analysis. *JMIR mHealth and uHealth*, 7, e13608.

Taubert, M., Watts, G., Boland, J. & Radbruch, L. 2014. Palliative social media. *BMJ Supportive & Palliative Care*, 4, 13–18.

United Nations: Department of Economic and Social Affairs 2023. World Social Report 2023: Leaving no One Behind in an Ageing World Website of the United Nations.

Volpi, E., Nazemi, R. & Fujita, S. 2004. Muscle tissue changes with aging. *Current Opinion in Clinical Nutrition & Metabolic Care*, 7, 405–410.

Waqar, M. A., Conright, K., Currie, D. R. & Cate, J. C. 2017. Technological advancements in pain management in the elderly population. *Using Technol. Improve Care Older Adults*, 124.

World Health Organization. 2024. *Ageing and health* [Online]. Website of the World Health Organization. Available: https://www.who.int/news-room/fact-sheets/detail/ageing-and-health [Accessed 24th March 2025].

Wrzesińska, N. 2015. The use of smart glasses in healthcare–review. *MEDtube Sci*, 31.

Yusif, S., Soar, J. & Hafeez-Baig, A. 2016. Older people, assistive technologies, and the barriers to adoption: A systematic review. *International journal of medical informatics*, 94, 112–116.

6 The Use of Technology to Provide Psychosocial Care in Palliative Care

6.1 The Challenge

People living with serious illness often experience psychological issues related to stress, anxiety and depression (Kredentser and Chochinov, 2020, Sultana et al., 2021). These problems might develop from diagnosis and can impact on personal and professional relationships (National Institute for Health and Clinical Excellence, 2004). Psychological wellbeing is influenced by both the external environment (e.g., family dynamics, cultural values and beliefs), and the internal environment (e.g., a person's thoughts, feelings, and behaviors) (Orenstein and Lewis, 2023).

Social support networks can positively influence wellbeing and quality-of-life (Berkman et al., 2000). Through these networks, patients can obtain emotional support from others, which is associated with better quality-of-life, reduced anxiety and depression (Bradley et al., 2018). The increasing use of technologies presents new opportunities for healthcare practitioners to provide psychosocial support to patients (Fig. 6.1).

6.2 What's in This Chapter?

This chapter considers how AgeTech can support psychosocial care for people living with terminal illness. Harry's persona illustrates how technologies can be used to provide a supportive social environment, which can encourage social connections, companionship and help to relieve some of the psychological burdens associated with serious illness. The chapter concludes with examples of digital interventions, which aim to encourage social interactions, which may positively impact mental well-being and quality-of-life.

A. C. Nwosu et al., *Technologies in Palliative Care for Older People*, Synthesis Lectures on Technology and Health, https://doi.org/10.1007/978-3-032-04277-4_6

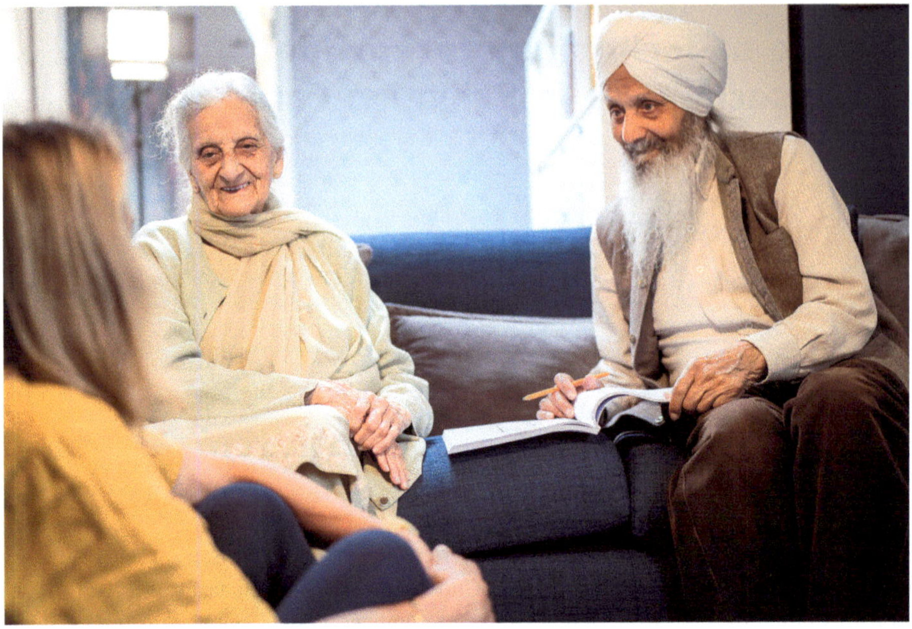

Fig. 6.1 *Credit* Peter Kindersley/aging better

6.3 Persona and Scenario—Harry

Persona: Harry is a 79-year-old man who lives alone on the outskirts of Birmingham, UK. He was diagnosed with COPD four years ago and following a hospital admission, two months ago, he was diagnosed with incurable lung cancer. His health is becoming progressively worse, meaning that he struggles to leave the house; he is now dependent on oxygen, and he is becoming increasingly short of breath on exertion. Harry has a portable oxygen cylinder but is wary of using it in public; he also worries that he will be unable to control his breathing if he were outside the house. Harry retired from his work as a bus driver aged 60, when his wife was diagnosed with breast cancer. Harry was able to support his wife's palliative care needs at home, until she was admitted to a local hospice to receive end-of-life care until she died. Harry has a son, a daughter-in-law and a granddaughter who live in Canada. Harry lives independently in his own home; he cooks his own meals and he manages his own personal hygiene needs. Harry has experienced increasing shortness of breath, meaning he was unable to clean his house. Therefore, Harry hired a cleaner, Janine, who comes once a week to clean his house for an hour. Janine also goes shopping for Harry and provides him with groceries on her weekly visits. Harry spends most of his time watching television or playing games on his tablet. Harry is very sociable; after his wife's death he became a member of a boules

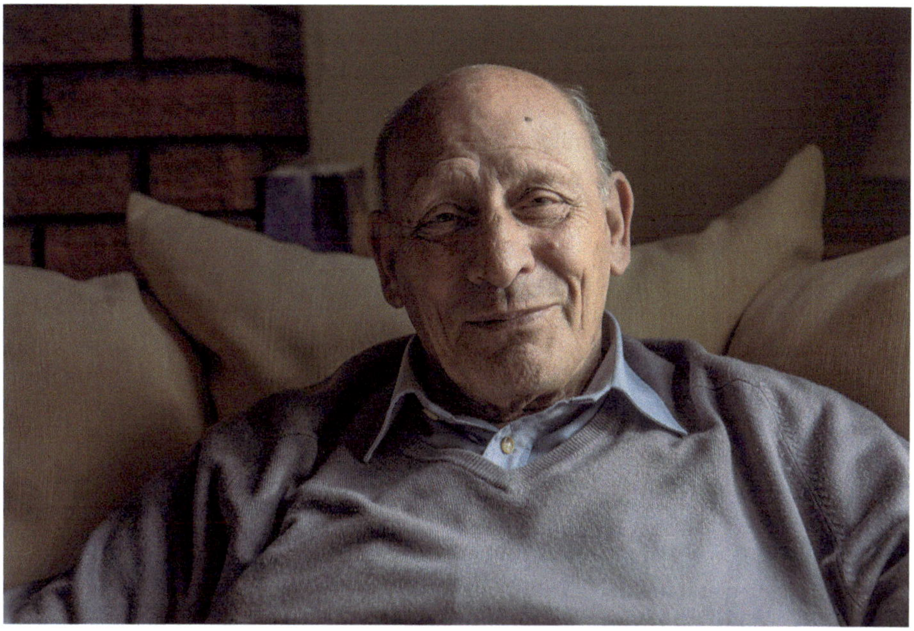

Fig. 6.2 *Credit* Mark Epstein/aging better

team and enjoys making friends. Harry often feels depressed that he is no longer able to attend social meetings with his friends because of his deteriorating health (Fig. 6.2).

Scenario: Harry's health has been deteriorating over the last six months, and he is now unable to do the activities he enjoys. Previously, when Harry was well, he visited his family in Canada and provided childcare of his granddaughter. He has been unable to travel to Canada because of his worsening breathlessness and concerns of the safety of travelling since the COVID-19 pandemic. Although he has weekly phone calls with his family, he misses seeing them and feels sad that he is not present to see his granddaughter grow. Harry feels lonely; the only person he now sees regularly is Janine (his cleaner), but he understands that she has limited time to spend at his house, and it is important that she has time to do her job. Harry's friends from the boules team contact him; however, their contact is infrequent, and Harry does not want to burden them with his feelings. Harry feels alone, and although the therapists at the COPD clinic encourage him to go out, his lack of confidence prevents this. Harry will often sit alone and cry, but he does not let anyone see this.

Solution: Technology can potentially be used to help Harry make social connections at home; however, it is important that Harry is confident to use these tools. During a visit, Janine spoke to Harry about the potential to use online platforms (such as, social media and gaming) to make social connections. Harry discovers a lung cancer support group through Facebook. He connects with others living with lung cancer and discovers that many are experiencing the same symptoms as he is. Through the group, he is introduced to games such as scrabble and jigsaw puzzles, which he uses to connect and play with others.

During a phone call to his family, Harry suggests that they play some of these games together during the evenings and weekends. Harry has found that his granddaughter enjoys playing these games, and she regularly sends him messages to ask when he is free to play. Harry decided to create a WhatsApp group with his friends from the boules club. Harry and his friends regularly send messages with jokes and photos, and he enjoys seeing pictures of the competition on the boules green. With support and a connection with his from the boules club, both in person and online, Harry's mood improves. He feels more confident, and happier, using the technology to tackle his loneliness.

6.4 Technologies to Support Psychosocial Care

Technologies are increasingly used to support social connections (Sen et al., 2022). When supporting communities, 'digital' might therefore, be considered an important, new dimension of wellbeing (Norris, 2024). The number of people using video communication platforms (for example Zoom, Microsoft Teams, Facetime and WhatsApp) to connect with families and friends has increased following the COVID-19 pandemic (Pitsillides and Wallace, 2021). These platforms have been used to provide support for symptom control, for example breathlessness groups, and peer support for people with serious illness (Stanley et al., 2024). Social media has been used to develop communities of support to reduce loneliness and exclusion in older people; however, it is important that older people are supported to use technology well to achieve this potential benefit. One initiative which seeks to address digital exclusion amongst older people is 'The Digital Champion Program 2022–2026' of Age UK (https://www.ageuk.org.uk/our-impact/programs/digital-skills/digital-champions) (detailed in Box 6.1).

Box 6.1

The digital champion program 2022–2026 (Age UK).

https://www.ageuk.org.uk/our-impact/programs/digital-skills/digital-champions/.

The digital champion program is an initiative developed by Age UK, a charity dedicated to helping older people. This program looks to tackle digital exclusion in older people by improving their digital skills. The program will train volunteers who will inspire and motivate others to get online, encouraging and supporting them to develop their digital skills and confidence. The digital champion program will provide both training, and equipment to those who need it, to help older people feel less isolated and more socially connected.

6.5 Use of Gaming Play for Companionship

Gaming offers opportunities for social connection, with studies demonstrating positive outcomes including social connectedness, improved knowledge and problem-solving skills and increased physical health (Dobbins et al., 2020). Whilst experiencing these positive outcomes, there is also evidence to suggest that online game playing amongst older people can improve quality-of-life, improve mood and reduce depression (Seah et al., 2018; Allaire et al., 2013). Some online games offer ways to play games independently (against a computer), to join online gaming communities or to invite friends to play (as illustrated in Box 6.2).

Box 6.2
Words With Friends 2, by Zynga.

Zynga is an American based company who have been developing online social games since 2007, with a mission to connect the world through games. 'Words with friends 2' is an online word game which allows players to challenge their own knowledge and skills in daily challenges and solo games, or to engage with multiplayer games as part of an online community. Players are also able to invite friends to join them in playing.

6.6 The Role of Robots

Robots have been used within healthcare to support social interaction (Nwosu et al., 2019), particularly in people with cognitive impairment (Huschilt and Clune, 2012; Darragh et al., 2017). Some of the benefits to using robots include joy, social influence and companionship. However, barriers exist for measingfulful use, which include negative societal attitudes towards robots, prohibitive cost, and a variety of technical and practical issues (Andtfolk et al., 2022). Robots show promise for the future and have the potential to provide companionship. One example of the use of robots for companionship is Paro the seal (described in Box 6.3).

Box 6.3

Paro the seal.

Paro the seal is a plush robotic seal created by Takanori Shibata, a robotics engineer. It was designed for use amongst Japan's aging population with an aim to provide similar benefits to a real pet such as reducing anxiety, encouraging social interaction and providing companionship. This model has been used worldwide in care homes and hospitals where there are factors preventing visits from live companion pets. Paro is programmed to respond to users with a range of emotions. Paro can learn its own name and respond to individuals based on how they stroke it; helping to build a companion relationship.

6.7 The Role of Technology in Spiritual Care

The social distancing enforced by the COVID-19 pandemic caused an evolution of many of traditional societal rituals, where people used technology to maintain social connection (Pitsillides and Wallace, 2021). A variety of devices (e.g., tablets and mobile phones), alongside communication platforms (e.g., WhatsApp and Zoom) have been used to help support spiritual care (Lazzarino and Papadopoulos, 2023).

6.8 Psychological Support

Mindfulness applications provide users with a method to relieve symptoms of stress, depression and anxiety (Gál et al., 2021). Several apps exist to help manage psychological issues, and provide users with the opportunity to access support and resources (Mikolasek et al., 2021). Many of these apps use a variety of different techniques to help users develop methods to manage their mental wellbeing (as described in Box 6.4).

Box 6.4

Healthy Minds Program App.

The healthy minds program app provides a framework to guide users through four pillars of training the mind: Awareness, connection, insight, purpose. The app includes a variety of techniques including podcasts, seated and active meditations and a healthy mind report which aim to train the user in strengthening their own wellbeing.

6.9 Artificial Intelligence Applications in Psychosocial Care

AI has been used to provide companionship, via virtual partners, life coaches or romantic partners (Pan and Mou, 2024). Replika (https://replika.com) is an AI-powered chatbot companion, developed in by Luca Inc, in San Francisco and launched in 2017 (Luka Inc, 2025). Replika learns to talk by studying billions of examples of human speech, generating a response that is realistic to human conversation. AI companions, like Replika, can offer valuable emotional support and companionship for those who feel isolated or lonely. They can provide a non-judgmental space for individuals to express their feelings, which can be helpful for those struggling with mental health issues like anxiety or depression. AI companions can also offer round-the-clock assistance to elderly or disabled individuals, providing both practical reminders and companionship to help reduce feelings of isolation and improve overall well-being (Pan and Mou, 2024).

However, the use of AI technology introduces a range of practical, psychological, and ethical challenges. One major concern is the potential impact on human relationships, as developing emotional connections with AI could lead individuals to prioritize digital interactions over face-to-face relationships. This shift may weaken human-to-human bonds and alter the dynamics of social interaction, as people become more reliant on virtual companions rather than engaging with others in the real world (Damiano and Dumouchel, 2018).

Additionally, this technology could influence the way people experience and process grief (Hollanek and Nowaczyk-Basińska, 2024). For those who have lost loved ones, AI's role in preserving and commemorating memories may change the way we remember the deceased, perhaps leading to new methods of mourning or altering traditional grieving practices. The emotional attachment individuals form with virtual agents poses a unique challenge: when these digital entities are 'deleted' or cease to exist, it may evoke strong emotional reactions (Stokes, 2015). The 'death' of a virtual companion could trigger feelings of loss, like those associated with the death of a real person, complicating how individuals manage their emotions and navigate the grieving process. This complexity of technology, emotions, and ethics raises important questions about the future of human relationships and the emotional landscape in an increasingly digital world.

6.10 Key Initiatives

The increasing use of AgeTech provides new opportunities to support psychosocial well-being. The initiative outlined below highlights how technology can be used to relieve psychosocial burden.

NHS England talking therapies for anxiety and depression.

'Talking Therapies, for anxiety and depression' was developed by the UK National Health Service to improve access to psychological therapies for depression and anxiety. Therapies are evidence based and tailored to individual needs. Many users choose to have therapy remotely (via video platform, telephone or text talk). During the program, patients are also encouraged to access digital treatment via the internet. Alongside a trained therapist, the use of digital treatment encourages patients to learn about managing their psychological symptoms and is available at any time of the day.

6.11 Find Out More

The digital champion program 2022–2026 (Age UK).

https://www.ageuk.org.uk/our-impact/programs/digital-skills/digital-champions.

Zynga Words with friends 2.

https://www.zynga.com/games/words-with-friends-2/.

Paro the seal.

https://www.paroseal.co.uk/.

Healthy Minds Program.

https://hminnovations.org/meditation-app.

NHS England talking therapies for anxiety and depression.

https://www.england.nhs.uk/mental-health/adults/nhs-talking-therapies/.

References

Allaire, J. C., Mclaughlin, A. C., Trujillo, A., Whitlock, L. A., Laporte, L. & Gandy, M. 2013. Successful aging through digital games: Socioemotional differences between older adult gamers and Non-gamers. *Computers in Human Behavior*, 29, 1302–1306.

Andtfolk, M., Nyholm, L., Eide, H. & Fagerström, L. 2022. Humanoid robots in the care of older persons: A scoping review. *Assistive Technology*, 34, 518–526.

Berkman, L. F., Glass, T., Brissette, I. & Seeman, T. E. 2000. From social integration to health: Durkheim in the new millennium. *Soc Sci Med*, 51, 843–57.

Bradley, N., Lloyd-Williams, M. & Dowrick, C. 2018. Effectiveness of palliative care interventions offering social support to people with life-limiting illness—A systematic review. *European Journal of Cancer Care*, 27, e12837.

Damiano, L. & Dumouchel, P. 2018. Anthropomorphism in human-robot co-evolution. Front Psychol, 9 (MAR), 1–9.

Darragh, M., Ahn, H. S., Macdonald, B., Liang, A., Peri, K., Kerse, N. & Broadbent, E. 2017. Homecare Robots to Improve Health and Well-Being in Mild Cognitive Impairment and Early Stage Dementia: Results From a Scoping Study. *J Am Med Dir Assoc*, 18, 1099.e1–1099.e4.

Dobbins, S., Hubbard, E., Flentje, A., Dawson-Rose, C. & Leutwyler, H. 2020. Play provides social connection for older adults with serious mental illness: A grounded theory analysis of a 10-week exergame intervention. *Aging Ment Health*, 24, 596–603.

Gál, É., Ştefan, S. & Cristea, I. A. 2021. The efficacy of mindfulness meditation apps in enhancing users' well-being and mental health related outcomes: a meta-analysis of randomized controlled trials. *Journal of Affective Disorders*, 279, 131–142.

Hollanek, T. & Nowaczyk-Basińska, K. 2024. Griefbots, Deadbots, Postmortem Avatars: on Responsible Applications of Generative AI in the Digital Afterlife Industry. *Philosophy & Technology*, 37, 1–22.

Huschilt, J. & Clune, L. 2012. The use of socially assistive robots for dementia care. *J Gerontol Nurs*, 38, 15–9.

Lazzarino, R. & Papadopoulos, I. 2023. Earbuds, smartphones, and music. Spiritual care and existential changes in COVID-19 times. *Social Theory & Health*, 21, 247–266.

Luka Inc. 2025. *Replika* [Online]. Available: https://replika.com/ [Accessed 25th March 2025].

Maia S. Kredentser, PH.D., & Harvey Max Chochinov, M.D., PH.D. 2020. Psychotherapeutic Considerations for Patients With Terminal Illness. *American Journal of Psychotherapy*, 73, 137–143.

Mikolasek, M., Witt, C. M. & Barth, J. 2021. Effects and implementation of a mindfulness and relaxation app for patients with cancer: Mixed methods feasibility study. *JMIR cancer*, 7, e16785.

National Institute for Health and Clinical Excellence. 2004. *Improving supportive and palliative care for adults with cancer* [Online]. Available: https://www.nice.org.uk/guidance/csg4 [Accessed 28.03.2023 2023].

Norris, J. 2024. *P-32 The wellbeing hub – reimagining wellbeing services.* https://doi.org/10.1136/spcare-2024-HUNC.53.

Nwosu, A. C., Sturgeon, B., Mcglinchey, T., Goodwin, C. D., Behera, A., Mason, S., Stanley, S. & Payne, T. R. 2019. Robotic technology for palliative and supportive care: Strengths, weaknesses, opportunities and threats. *Palliative Medicine*, 33, 1106–1113.

Orenstein, G. A. & Lewis, L. 2023. Eriksons Stages of Psychosocial Development. *StatPearls*. Treasure Island (FL): StatPearls Publishing.

Pan, S. & Mou, Y. 2024. Constructing the meaning of human–AI romantic relationships from the perspectives of users dating the social chatbot Replika. *Personal Relationships.*

Pitsillides, S. & Wallace, J. 2021. Physically distant but socially connected: Streaming funerals, memorials and ritual design during COVID-19. *Death, grief and loss in the context of COVID-19*, 60–76.

Seah, E. T. W., Kaufman, D., Sauvé, L. & Zhang, F. 2018. Play, Learn, Connect: Older Adults' Experience With a Multiplayer, Educational, Digital Bingo Game. *Journal of Educational Computing Research*, 56, 675–700.

Sen, K., Prybutok, G. & Prybutok, V. 2022. The use of digital technology for social wellbeing reduces social isolation in older adults: A systematic review. *SSM Popul Health*, 17, 101020.

Stanley, S., Finucane, A., Thompson, A. & Nwosu, A. C. 2024. How can technology be used to support communication in palliative care beyond the covid-19 pandemic: a mixed-methods national survey of palliative care healthcare professionals. *BMC palliative care*, 23, 40.

Stokes, P. 2015. Deletion as second death: The moral status of digital remains. *Ethics and Information Technology*, 17, 237–248.

Sultana, A., Tasnim, S., Sharma, R., Pawar, P., Bhattcharya, S. & Hossain, M. M. 2021. Psychosocial challenges in palliative care: Bridging the gaps using digital health. *Indian journal of palliative care*, 27, 442.

Coordination of Clinical Care

7

7.1 The Challenge

It is important that decision-makers coordinate the services needed to provide holistic palliative care for older people, which addresses their physical, emotional, and psychosocial needs (Firth et al., 2025). People may require palliative care in different settings, such as the home, hospital and hospice. Therefore, it is important that care providers have the necessary resources to deliver timely support for patients wherever they are (Chan et al., 2021).

Coordinating palliative care services for individuals can be challenging due to many factors, such as the medical complexity, limited resources and the challenge of providing care across settings, which lack interoperable ICT infrastructure (Jones et al., 2023). Technology-based solutions offer opportunities to improve clinical care coordination (Petrova et al., 2018). For example, digital technologies (such as smartphones, wearables and sensors) offer tools to facilitate early diagnosis, screening of illness, self-care, therapy and remote monitoring of healthcare needs (Nwosu et al., 2022).

7.2 What's in This Chapter

This chapter outlines the technologies and approaches available for healthcare professionals to coordinate the medical management of an older person with palliative care needs. Some technologies described may be relevant to the different healthcare needs that people encounter throughout their illness; however, this chapter focuses on frail individuals who are likely to deteriorate and require end-of-life care. As illustrated in Emma's story

A. C. Nwosu et al., *Technologies in Palliative Care for Older People*, Synthesis Lectures on Technology and Health, https://doi.org/10.1007/978-3-032-04277-4_7

below, we demonstrate how AgeTech can be used to coordinate palliative care decision-making for an older person, by using technology to support diagnosis, monitoring and data analysis.

7.3 Persona and Scenario

Persona: Emma is a 76-year-old woman who lives in a bungalow in a densely populated neighbourhood in Boston, USA. Emma is a retired accountant, and she lives alone. Emma was the main caregiver for her husband, who recently died following a long illness. Emma has several medical problems, including COPD (a chronic breathing problem affecting the lungs) and osteoarthritis. Emma's activities have been severely limited due to her illnesses. For example, it is painful for Emma to walk becuase of her arthritis and she is always breathless due to her COPD. Emma was previously very active, enjoying walking and gardening; however, she now does fewer physical activities. Emma now prefers less physical hobbies, such as reading, solving puzzles, and receiving the occasional visit from her neighbors (Fig. 7.1).

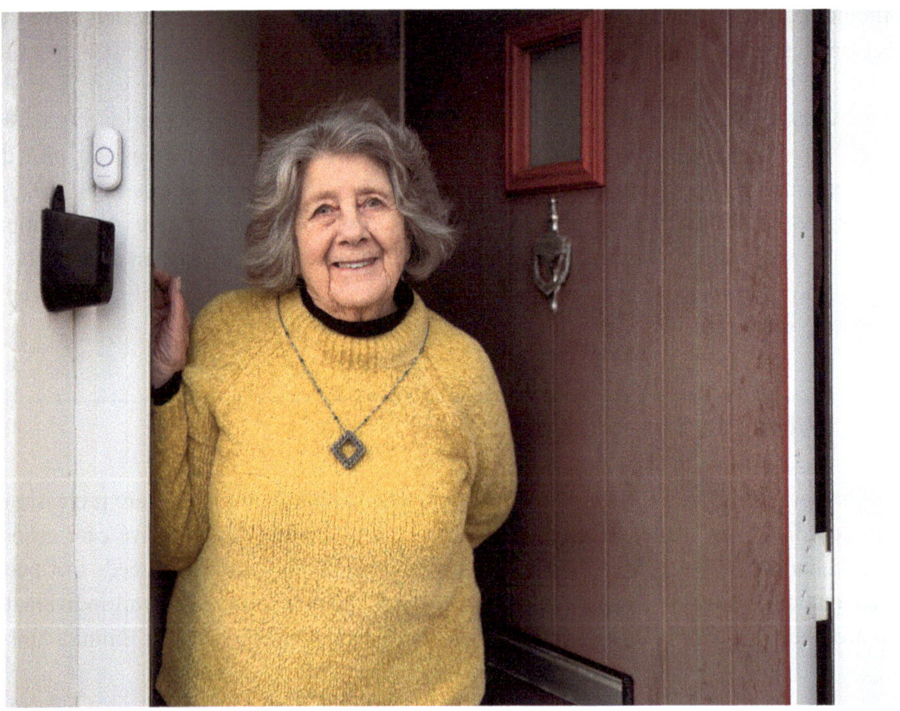

Fig. 7.1 *Credit* Mark Epstein/aging better

Scenario: Emma's family live in different places in the world; her children live in Texas (USA), London (UK) and Vancouver (Canada). Her children are worried that Emma is becoming frailer and will become unable to care for herself at home. Emma wants to increase her independence and physical activity, but she is worried about falling and being unable contact people if she needs help. Emma wants practical solutions to help her live at home independently and to obtain support when needed.

Solution: Emma wants more options to assist communications with her friends and family. She wants more control of her healthcare and she wants the ability to contact her medical team, to ask for help, when she is unwell. Emma's children advise her to use technology to support her activities of daily living. Her children provide Emma with a smartwatch, a smartphone, a tablet, and an AI home smart speaker. Also, her children install a smart home monitoring system (using sensor-based technologies and trackers) to monitor Emma's activity around the house. These monitoring devices collect and analyze Emma's data in real-time, to provide her (and her family) with treatment recommendations and alert care providers to changes in her routine.

Emma has embraced these technologies, as she uses her mobile devices for virtual consultations with her medical team. Each day, Emma uses her smartwatch to record her oxygen saturations, heart-rate and sleep quality. Emma's smartwatch communicates with her smart home system (which includes sensors in her bedroom and kitchen), that alerts her family (and healthcare provider) if Emma falls or if a worrying change in her normal routine is detected. Emma uses her smart speaker to manage her social media profiles, to automate devices and to make video calls with her friends and family. Emma is happy with the new skills she has developed, and she believes that her AgeTech tools have helped her to improve her digital literacy. Emma's children are impressed by her improved confidence, independence and social connections, which they feel is due to her use of AgeTech.

7.4 Technology to Coordinate Care for Older People with Palliative Care Problems

Diagnosis and screening

Technology can be used to support diagnosis and early detection of illnesses. For example, initiatives like MyWear (a smart garment that continuously monitors and collects physiological data) can analyze a user's muscle activity, stress levels, and heart rate variations (and subsequently send this data to cloud storage) (Sethuraman et al., 2021). Another example is the use of an earbud, which can potentially detect neurodegenerative diseases by continuously monitoring brain activity and measuring lactate concentrations in sweat (Xu et al., 2023). Similarly, many smartwatches (e.g. the Apple watch) provide a range of biometric assessments to support health management, such as electrocardiogram heartrate monitoring, oxygen saturation, and sending distress messages (e.g. a nominated person or emergency services) if a fall is detected (Köhler et al., 2024; Nwosu et al., 2018).

Self-care and management

Older people can access their electronic medical records and use digital tools to self-manage their health. For example, in England most patients (> 81%) have access to their electronic medical record, using their own computer or mobile device (NHS England, 2023). Patients may use video communication software and messaging services for remote consultations with their healthcare providers. An example is the Chain SMS system by Accurx (a British healthcare software company), which is used by over 90% of primary care clinics in England for remote consultations (Box 7.1). During the COVID-19 pandemic, the Accurx system integrated videoconferencing software and text-messaging capabilities, enabling direct communication between patients and healthcare professionals. Other examples of video communication technology include the 'Resilience Lab', which offers an online service for matching clients with therapists to receive online counselling sessions (Box 7.2).

Box 7.1

Accurx's (a British healthcare software company) main product is Chain SMS, a messaging program used by doctor surgeries to communicate with patients. The program runs on desktop computers and integrates with electronic health care record systems. Accurx sends SMS text messages to patients to facilitate communication with their medical practice. Since the COVID-19 pandemic in the UK, Accurx integrated a videotelephony system into their SMS systems, to support healthcare professionals to use the system to conduct remote consultations.

Box 7.2

Resilience Lab (https://www.resiliencelab.us/) is an American company which build a bridge between academic training and real-world experiences within the mental health field, to address the problem of a shortage of well-trained therapists and a lack of diversity among clinicians. The New York-based company has three product and service offerings: Resilience Lab, Resilience Institute and Resilience Dashboard. The Resilience Lab is an in-person and online service that matches clients with clinicians. Clients use the company's website to connect to therapists and participate in either in-person, telehealth or hybrid sessions (Fig. 7.2).

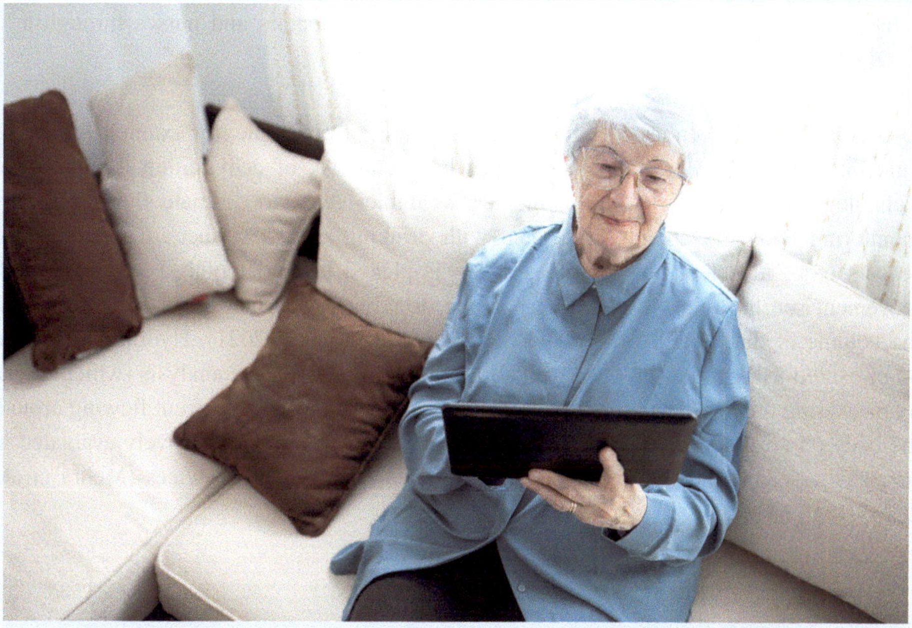

Fig. 7.2 *Credit* Gligatron/Shutterstock

Monitoring and assessment

Previous studies demonstrate how sensor-based systems and internet-connected devices (IoT) in home environments (i.e. a smart home) can use remote monitoring and automation of appliances (such as lighting and heating) to support care for people experiencing a decline in their physical function (Haghi et al., 2017; Liu et al., 2016). Examples include Atrium Health (USA's largest hospital at home provider (Swick et al., 2022)) who have formed a collaboration with Best Buy (an American consumer electronics retailer) to use technology to remotely monitor users and analyze the data to inform personalized care at home (Hudson, 2023) (Box 7.3).

Box 7.3

Atrium Health (https://atriumhealth.org/) is the USA's largest hospital-at-home provider, allowing patients with certain medical conditions to receive hospital-level care in the comfort of their own home. Atrium Health has partnered with Best Buy Health to enhance the patient experience, by using specially trained 'Geek Squad' agents, who set up the technology in the person's home. The devices remotely monitor the person's heart rate, blood oxygen level, or other vitals. The technology platform then securely shares the data with doctors and nurses through a telemedicine hub.

Technology has been used to monitor hydration in older people; for example, to record fluid intake in older care home residents who are at risk of dehydration. Examples of technologies to monitor hydration include wearables (e.g., to estimate fluid intake by monitoring body movements associated with drinking), smart surfaces with embedded sensors (e.g., to detect how often as a cup is picked up and replaced), cameras with movement sensors (e.g., to observe someone drinking), and smart cups (e.g., to record the volume of fluid drank from a specific cup) (Cohen et al., 2021). Hydration can also be measured using a non-invasive technology called bioimpedance analysis (which works by measuring the resistance to a low frequency, painless, electrical current flowing around the body (Nwosu et al., 2014)). Bioimpedance analysis has been extensively evaluated in scientific research and is increasingly incorporated into wearable devices (Mehra et al., 2024) (Fig. 7.3).

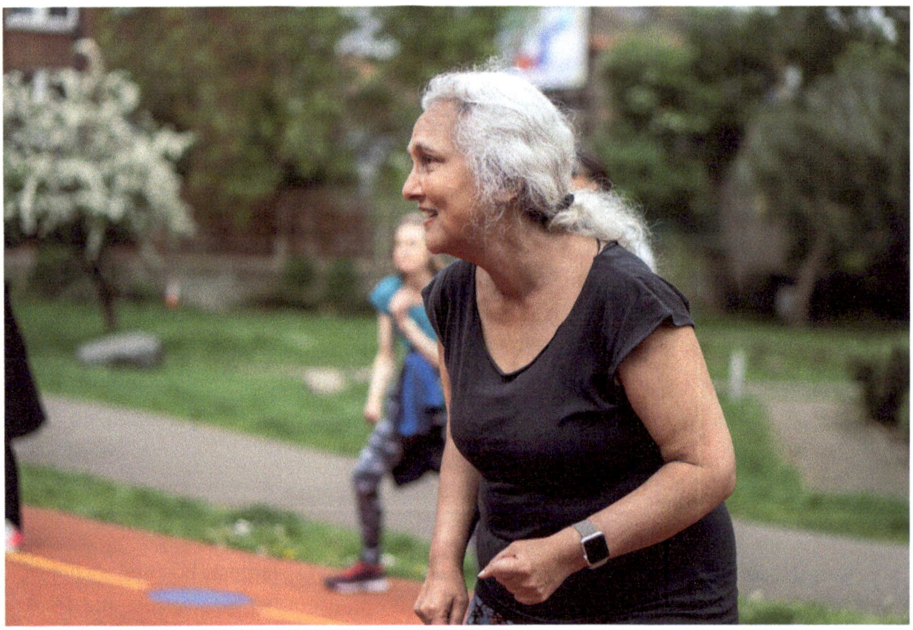

Fig. 7.3 *Credit* Elliot Manches/aging better

7.5 Artificial Intelligence Applications to Coordinate Palliative Care Services for Older People

Howz (a company in the United Kingdom) have developed a smart home monitoring system, using a combination of sensors and an app, to passively collect data from the home. The Howz smart home monitoring system works through a combination of the Howz app and sensors installed in the house of the older person. This includes physiological devices used by the resident (thermometer, oximeter, a smart tablet), environmental sensors (a smart plug used to monitor electrical usage from appliances like kettles, a door sensor to track door opening, a motion sensor to assess movement and a wireless hub). The Howz system continuously collects and analyses sensor data, to establish a normal pattern of the resident's behavior, to detect real-time problems requiring intervention. For example, data showing reduced electricity uses from a kettle, reduced movement on the monitor sensors, and erratic heart monitoring may indicate that the resident is unwell and needs help. The Howz system can alert family members (and healthcare professionals) to changes of the resident, to help determine what support is needed. Evaluations of the Howz system reports benefits for people with stroke (Rogerson et al., 2020) and dementia (Kent Surrey Sussex Academic Health Science Network, 2021),with further economic benefits demonstrated due to reductions in emergency medical admissions (Fig. 7.4).

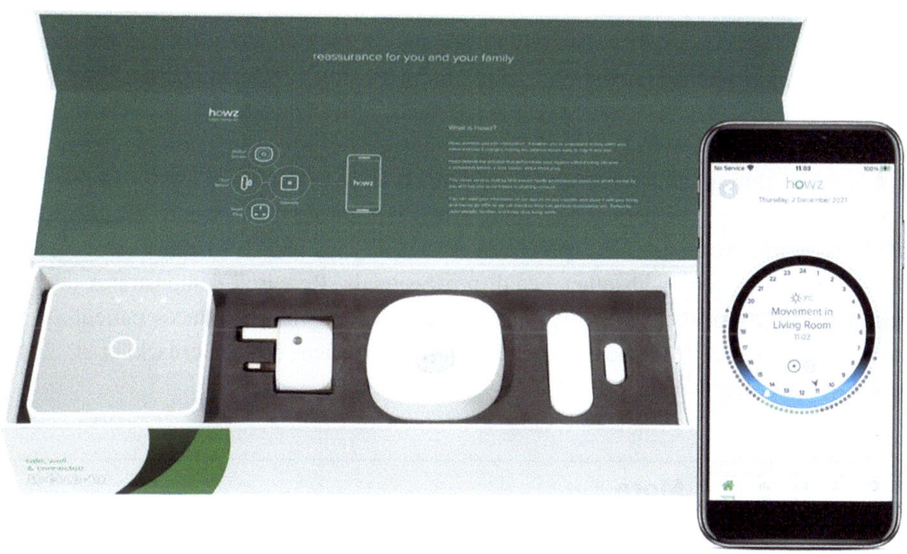

Fig. 7.4 The Howz home monitoring system consists of a motion sensor, a door sensor, a smart plug and a gateway device to analyse the data. *Credit* Howz

7.6 Key Initiatives

Electronic Palliative Care Coordinating Systems (EPaCCS) in England

Electronic Palliative Care Coordination Systems (EPaCCS) are an England based initiative to enable advance care planning and improve communication and coordination at the end-of-life (Petrova et al., 2018). EPaCCS are electronic registers or tools and processes for sharing data, which aim to enable access to information about dying patients. EPaCCS exist in different English health and local government authorities to enable care records to be coordinated electronically. Practically, this involves a shared electronic record between different healthcare providers, professionals, and agencies, which allow the record to be shared, viewed and updated by professionals working in any setting where the individual receives care. EPaCCS offer practical benefits, resulting from improved coordination of care and communication, between professionals involved in a patient's end-of-life care.

Examples of EPaCCS are the London 'MyWishes Care' services (https://mywishes.care), where information about a person's care preferences are stored alongside other information, such as diagnosis, medical details, resuscitation status, medications and emergency management plans. The care plan can then be shared with all the urgent care services, including out of hours medical services, the ambulance and the emergency departments.

Serious Illness Care Program

The Serious Illness Care Program (SICP) is a system-based approach for improving serious illness care, was developed at Ariadne Labs, Boston, USA (Bernacki et al., 2015a). The Serious Illness Conversation Guide provides a framework for physicians, nurses, social workers, chaplains, allied health professionals, and other clinicians to explore topics that are crucial to gaining a full understanding about (and honoring) what is most important to patients. The SICP involves integration with hospital Electronic Patient Records (EPR) systems, to create clear processes to identify patients and document important conversations to share with other health professionals. Research demonstrates the SICP results in early (and better quality) conversations about illness, reduces patient anxiety, improves experience for patients and clinicians, and reduces costs (Bernacki et al., 2015b; McGlinchey et al., 2019).

7.7 Find Out More

Petrova, M., Riley, J., Abel, J. and Barclay, S., 2018. Crash course in EPaCCS (Electronic Palliative Care Coordination Systems): 8 years of successes and failures in patient data sharing to learn from. BMJ supportive & palliative care, 8(4), pp.447–455.

https://spcare.bmj.com/content/8/4/447.

References

Bernacki, R., Hutchings, M., Vick, J., Smith, G., Paladino, J., Lipsitz, S., Gawande, A. A. & Block, S. D. 2015a. Development of the Serious Illness Care Program: a randomised controlled trial of a palliative care communication intervention. *BMJ open,* 5, e009032.

Bernacki, R., Paladino, J., Lamas, D., Hutchings, M., Lakin, J., Neville, B. A., Lipsitz, S. R., Gawande, A. & Block, S. 2015b. Delivering more, earlier, and better goals-of-care conversations to seriously ill oncology patients. American Society of Clinical Oncology.

Chan, H. Y.-L., Chung, C. K.-M., Tam, S. S.-C. & Chow, R. S.-K. 2021. Community palliative care services on addressing physical and psychosocial needs in people with advanced illness: a prospective cohort study. *BMC Palliative Care,* 20, 1–8.

Cohen, R., Fernie, G. & Roshan Fekr, A. 2021. Fluid intake monitoring systems for the elderly: A review of the literature. *Nutrients,* 13, 2092.

Firth, A. M., Goodrich, J., Gaczkowska, I., Harding, R., Murtagh, F. E. & Evans, C. J. 2025. Community out-of-hours palliative care–'It'sa patchwork of services': A qualitative study exploring care provision. *Palliative Medicine,* 39, 245–255.

Haghi, M., Thurow, K. & Stoll, R. 2017. Wearable Devices in Medical Internet of Things: Scientific Research and Commercially Available Devices. *Healthc Inform Res,* 23, 4–15.

Hudson, C. 2023. Best Buy Health leans into at-home care through large provider deals. *Modern Healthcare,* 53, 0008–0008.

Jones, R., Dale, J. & Macartney, J. 2023. Challenges experienced by GPs when providing palliative care in the UK: a systematic qualitative literature review. *BJGP open,* 7.

Kent Surrey Sussex Academic Health Science Network 2021. Technology Integrated Health Managament (TIHM): Health economic evaluation.

Köhler, C., Bartschke, A., Fürstenau, D., Schaaf, T. & Salgado-Baez, E. 2024. The Value of Smartwatches in the Health Care Sector for Monitoring, Nudging, and Predicting: Viewpoint on 25 Years of Research. *Journal of Medical Internet Research,* 26, e58936.

Liu, L., Stroulia, E., Nikolaidis, I., Miguel-Cruz, A. & Rios Rincon, A. 2016. Smart homes and home health monitoring technologies for older adults: A systematic review. *Int J Med Inform,* 91, 44–59.

Mcglinchey, T., Mason, S., Coackley, A., Roberts, A., Maguire, M., Sanders, J., Maloney, F., Block, S., Ellershaw, J. & Kirkbride, P. 2019. Serious illness care Programme UK: assessing the 'face validity', applicability and relevance of the serious illness conversation guide for use within the UK health care setting. *BMC health services research,* 19, 1–9.

Mehra, A., Starkoff, B. E. & Nickerson, B. S. 2024. The evolution of bioimpedance analysis: From traditional methods to wearable technology. *Nutrition,* 112601.

NHS England. 2023. *Access to patient records through the NHS App* [Online]. NHS England. Available: https://transform.england.nhs.uk/information-governance/guidance/access-to-patient-records-through-the-nhs-app/#:~:text=You%20have%20a%20legal%20right,practice%20to%20provide%20the%20information [Accessed 6th June 2024].

Nwosu, A., Mayland, C., Varro, A. & Ellershaw, J. 2014. The assessment of hydration in advanced cancer patients using bioelectrical impedance analysis. *BMJ Support Palliat Care,* 4 Suppl 1, A3.

Nwosu, A. C., Mcglinchey, T., Sanders, J., Stanley, S., Palfrey, J., Lubbers, P., Chapman, L., Finucane, A. & Mason, S. 2022. Identification of digital health priorities for palliative care research: modified delphi study. *JMIR aging,* 5, e32075.

Nwosu, A. C., Quinn, C., Samuels, J., Mason, S. & Payne, T. R. 2018. Wearable smartwatch technology to monitor symptoms in advanced illness. *BMJ supportive & palliative care,* 8, 237–237.

Petrova, M., Riley, J., Abel, J. & Barclay, S. 2018. Crash course in EPaCCS (Electronic Palliative Care Coordination Systems): 8 years of successes and failures in patient data sharing to learn from. *BMJ supportive & palliative care,* 8**,** 447–455.

Rogerson, L., Burr, J. & Tyson, S. 2020. The feasibility and acceptability of smart home technology using the Howz system for people with stroke. *Disability and Rehabilitation: Assistive Technology.*

Sethuraman, S. C., Kompally, P., Mohanty, S. P. & Choppali, U. 2021. MyWear: A novel smart garment for automatic continuous vital monitoring. *IEEE Transactions on Consumer Electronics,* 67**,** 214–222.

Swick, M., Mook, P. J. & Mcdonald, S. 2022. For All: Atrium Health Efforts Create a More Diverse, Inclusive Culture. *Nurse Leader,* 20**,** 336–339.

Xu, Y., de la Paz, E., Paul, A., Mahato, K., Sempionatto, J. R., Tostado, N., Lee, M., Hota, G., Lin, M. & Uppal, A. 2023. In-ear integrated sensor array for the continuous monitoring of brain activity and of lactate in sweat. *Nature Biomedical Engineering,* 7**,** 1307–1320.

8 Technology to Support Care at the End-of-Life

8.1 The Challenge

Technology can help healthcare professionals to provide end-of-life care to people who are dying (Nwosu et al., 2022). Examples of technological innovation in end-of-life care were evident during the COVID-19 pandemic, where many healthcare services incorporated technological tools to deliver palliative care services. Beyond the pandemic, it is important to ensure that AgeTech is used meaningfully, to provide person-centered care to older people who are dying (Stanley et al., 2024).

8.2 What's in This Chapter?

This chapter considers how digital technologies can support care at the end-of-life using the persona of June. We also explore how technologies can support documentation of care preferences, support digital legacy planning and provide bereavement support. The chapter concludes with some examples of digital health interventions, which potentially can be used to support end-of-life care.

8.3 Persona and Scenario—June

Persona: June is a 60-year-old woman living in Northern Ireland (UK). She was recently diagnosed with stage 4 metastatic bowel cancer. June is a grandmother to two children: Lily (age 6) and Max (age 8), who are cared for by their mother, Hannah (a lone parent). June frequently provides childcare, and she was very supportive of Hannah, Lily and

A. C. Nwosu et al., *Technologies in Palliative Care for Older People*, Synthesis Lectures on Technology and Health, https://doi.org/10.1007/978-3-032-04277-4_8

Max. June was admitted to a hospice to receive symptom management for pain. During the admission, June's condition worsened, and June's doctors told her that she will need to stay in the hospice to receive end-of-life care (due to the complexity of her clinical care needs). The hospice staff encouraged June's grandchildren to regularly visit June in the hospice, and the staff arranged activities to help her family to spend time together (e.g., family 'movie nights' where her family would watch movies together in June's room). June and Hannah were grateful to the staff for organizing these special family moments. Despite these activities, June was worried that her grandchildren would not remember her after her death, due to their young ages. June speaks to her daughter and the hospice staff about her concerns and she stated her intention to create an archive of sentimental items, to help Lily and Max remember special memories of June, when they see these items in the future (after her death) (Fig. 8.1).

Scenario: June's health has significantly worsened over the last few weeks. She lacks energy and spends a lot of time sleeping to conserve energy to play with her grandchildren when they visit the hospice. June enjoys spending time with her grandchildren, playing games and telling stories. Lily and Max enjoy sitting on June's bed, listening their grandmother share stories about her life as air hostess. Lily and Max are fascinated to learn about the places June has visited, and to hear her talk about her experiences. June shows her grandchildren pictures and video on her mobile phone (and social media

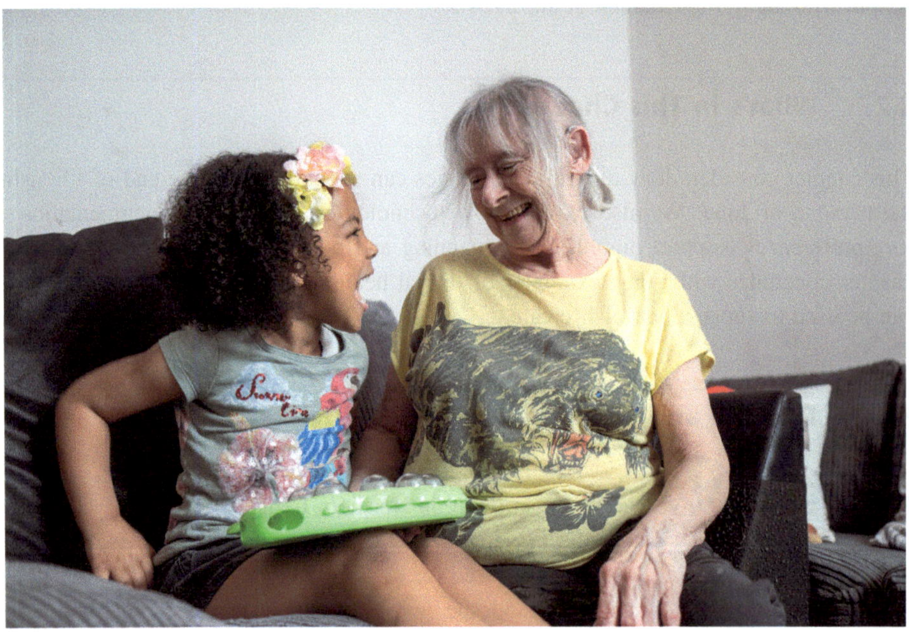

Fig. 8.1 *Credit* Elliot Manches/aging better

accounts) to add context to her stories. She is delighted to observe how the children enthusiastically respond to stories about her life.

June uses social media to record important events in her life, such as family celebrations. Over many years, June created a repository of memories in a digital format, by using her mobile phone to take taking photos and record videos. June's photos and videos are saved on her mobile phone and 'backed up' in the cloud (i.e., Google Photos). June enjoys listening to her music playlist on Spotify, and she often sings songs with her grandchildren, which have family significance. June often worries that these digital assets will be lost after her death; therefore, she wants to secure them for her grandchildren to cherish in the future.

Solution: June tells the hospice nurse that she is worried that grandchildren will not be able to access her digital photos and videos after her death. June has also told the nurse about her wish to leave personalized video messages for her grandchildren. The nurse provides advice to June on how she can arrange her digital life. June and the nurse talk about organizing legacy contacts for June's social media accounts. Through this process, June appoints her daughter (Hannah) to manage her Google and Facebook accounts after June's death; June provides Hannah with administrator access to ensure that her photos and videos are not lost. June and the nurse discuss options to download her favorite songs, create playlists for her grandchildren, and save the media to a portable storage drive. The nurse documents this conversation (and June's care preferences) on her EPR. Following the conversation, June begins to organize and archive important digital videos and photos on her phone, whilst deleting the content she does not want to leave behind following her death. June creates a 'Social Media Will' which outlines the arrangements she has made and describes her wishes for the management of her online accounts after she dies.

June speaks with the children's counselor based in the hospice, and she decides to create memory boxes. June records videos and voice notes for her grandchildren, which are stored on a portable storage drive in the box, alongside the physical photographs. June feels empowered and happy that she was able to curate, and create positive, mementoes for her grandchildren; she hopes these items will help with their grief following her death.

8.4 Technologies to Support Care at the End-of-Life

Technology use in palliative care is increasing, which creates new and innovative opportunities for healthcare professionals to support people at the end-of-life (Stanley et al., 2024). Furthermore, the increasing use of internet-enabled devices (and social media) creates opportunities for the public to create their own content on platforms such as TikTok (Ceci, 2022). The increasing volume of digital information about people means that digital preservation is becoming increasingly important, which has the potential to impact palliative care as people age with serious illness. One initiative looking to address preservation of digital assets is The Digital Preservation Coalition (https://www.dpconline.org) (detailed in Box 8.1).

Box 8.1
The Digital Preservation Coalition (https://www.dpconline.org/).

The digital preservation coalition is a global initiative which works with several organizations, aiming to bring about a sustainable future for digital assets. This initiative addresses issues around preservation of digital assets within organizations and provides practical case studies and guides for preserving personal digital collections.

8.5 Digital Legacy

A digital legacy is the digital information that is available about someone following their death. Someone's digital legacy is often shaped by interactions the person made and information that they created before they died. This might include their social media profiles, online conversations, photos, videos, gaming profiles and their website or blog. Someone's digital legacy can also be informed by content that is created or co-created by others. This may include interactions that have occurred on someone else's social media (The Digital Legacy Association, 2024).

Digital legacy has increasing societal importance for multifactorial reasons (Norris, 2024). For example, there is evolution in technological infrastructures (such as high-speed internet, mobile devices and portable photography), which has led to evolution of the way many people create and consume media. Increasingly, people are using digital devices to access, and store, digital information (e.g., digital photos, video and text notes), as opposed to physical media (e.g., written notes and photos) (Stanley et al., 2023) (Fig. 8.2).

In the scenario above, June's main device for capturing important moments in her life is her mobile device. The memories that she captures in the moment are not printed out and inserted into photo albums but instead they reside on her phone and across various social networks and online storage platforms (e.g. Google Photos).

For June, her mobile phone has replaced the function of her handwritten notebook, the analogue camera and video recorder. Instead of using physical DVDs and CDs to consume media, June streams media directly to her mobile device. June's story demonstrates that although behaviors such as listening to music, taking photos and consuming media have not changed, the interfaces some people use to access content continue to evolve.

Someone's digital legacy can be of great value to their friends and family after their death as this enables the living to continue to access the deceased person's digital media (such as, photos and videos, messages) to preserve their memory (Norris and Sofka, 2025). The living may find comfort by revisiting the deceased person's digital messages

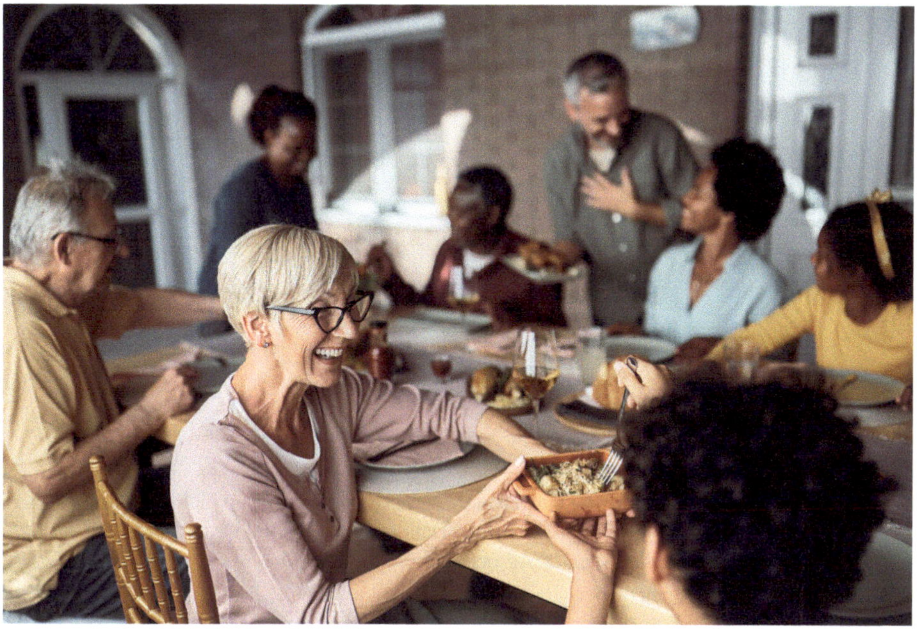

Fig. 8.2 *Credit* Drazen Zigic/Shutterstock

(such as a WhatsApp discussion thread) as a way to recall conversations held with, or about, that person when they were alive (Taubert et al., 2014). In addition to social networks, digital legacy is important to online communities, such as gaming (Stanley et al., 2023), fantasy football, music (Bellamy et al., 2013) and the arts (Suhardjono, 2023).

Healthcare decision makers and policymakers require appropriate tools, knowledge and information to support individuals (like June and those important to her) to ensure their digital assets are managed, according to their wishes, after death (Norris et al., 2022). The Digital Legacy Association, an organization that leads in managing digital assets after death, provides knowledge support for decision-makers and policymakers. Notably, the Digital Legacy Association produces an annual Digital Death Report, which provides important data international insights, to shape public discussion, education, practice and research (Norris and Sofka, 2025). June's strategy of using social/digital media to help her family remember her life is supported by the 2025 survey data, which shows bereaved respondents use these media for five main purposes: staying connected with the deceased, seeking grief support, supporting others, remembering the person, and fundraising (Fig. 8.3) (Norris and Sofka, 2025). The survey suggests that the public has a favorable view of using social media to remember the dead, with 58% of respondents describing social media use to share information relating to the death of a friend or family member as 'positive' (Norris and Sofka, 2025) (See in Sect. 10.13 for more information about the Digital Legacy Association and then Digital Death Report).

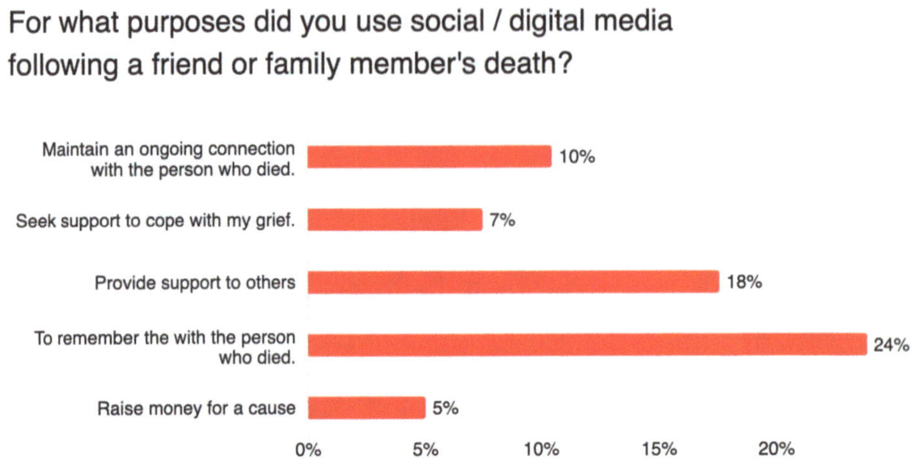

Fig. 8.3 A bar chart representing the reasons why bereaved people used social and/or digital media following the death of a friend of family member. Data from the Digital Death Report 2025 (Norris and Sofka, 2025). *Credit* Digital Legacy Association

8.6 Recording Care Preferences

It is important that people have the opportunity to a record their future care preferences (Malhotra et al., 2022). Studies show that people who document their future care preferences often experience better care, are more likely to have their wishes fulfilled and experience an improved quality-of-life (Easwar et al., 2022; Malhotra et al., 2022). People can record their care preferences through Advance Care Planning, which involves a patient discussing their care priorities with a healthcare professional. The healthcare professional will record this discussion in patient's medical record, on a document known as Advance Care Plan (ACP). The ACP is used to align medical decision making with the wishes and preferences of the patient. Traditionally, ACP documents are physical records, but are increasingly becoming digital records, incorporated in the EPR (Bernacki et al., 2015).

8.7 Technology to Support Care of the Dying

Technologies can be used to support care for dying people by facilitating pain and symptom control (Adam et al., 2018). Common examples include continuous subcutaneous infusion pumps, which are used to administer medications to people unable to take medications by mouth (Graham and Clark, 2005). Other technological techniques are available to manage pain; however, these procedures may not be suitable for those who are imminently dying (i.e. the last hours and days of life). For example, technological interventional pain management procedures includes intrathecal drug delivery systems (IDDS), which are implanted devices that deliver medication directly to the spinal fluid, providing sustained pain relief with lower doses of medication (Simpson, 2011). Minimally invasive interventional therapy procedures can manage pain; for example cementoplasties (e.g., kyphoplasty and vertebroplasty) involves the injection of cement into vertebral discs to stabilize and relieve pain caused by bone fractures (Hua et al., 2023). Cordotomy is a surgical procedure involving the interruption of pain pathways in the spinal cord, reducing pain sensation on one side of the body (Doyle et al., 2022). Radiofrequency ablation uses heat to destroy nerve tissue, mainly to manage for pain in cancer patients with bone metastases (Marchal et al., 2006). Neuromodulation uses technology to alter or modulate nerve activity, often through electrical or chemical stimulation. For example, spinal cord stimulation (SCS), involves implanting a device that sends electrical signals to the spinal cord to manage pain by interfering with pain signals travelling to the brain (Paolini et al., 2022).

Other technologies that can support the care of the dying include AI facial recognition technologies to help healthcare professionals assess pain in people unable to communicate (Brett and Severn, 2023). AI analytics of EPR data have been used to identify hospital patients with previously unidentified palliative care needs who may benefit from palliative care assessment and intervention (Avati et al., 2018; Durieux et al., 2022). Wearables and sensors have been used to assess sleep quality, falls and diagnose delirium and in the dying (Sandic Spaho et al., 2023). Non-invasive technologies like bioelectrical impedance analysis have been used to assess hydration in the dying (Nwosu et al., 2024), and bispectral index monitoring has been used assess cognition (Barbato, 2001). Biomarker research been used to estimate prognosis in dying patients by using a technique to detect chemicals in urine, which signify that the patient is in dying phase of their illness (Coyle et al., 2025) Personalized medicine (also known as precision medicine), is an emerging practice of medicine that uses a person's genetic profile to guide decisions made in regard to the prevention, diagnosis, and treatment of disease (Jackson and Chester, 2015). Personalized medicine offers opportunities to personalize palliative care therapies (such as pain) management according to an individual's genetic profile (Bruehl et al., 2013).

8.8 Communication During the Dying Phase

Communication technologies can support patients and caregivers receive appropriate information about dying phase. For example, websites of care providers and healthcare organizations can display relevant information for patients, caregivers and staff (Street et al., 2007). In care settings, digital information boards can be used to display information for the public (such as the location of wards, services and the names of healthcare staff) and staff (such as relevant patient information) (Favela et al., 2004; Hamidi et al., 2019). Email, mobile phone and SMS messages could be used more effectively to facilitate communication between healthcare professionals, patients and caregivers (Dash et al., 2016). Electronic palliative care coordination systems are important to ensure that healthcare professionals caring for the dying can access relevant information, including any changes to their preferences, wishes and personalized care plans (Petrova et al., 2018). One example of how this information could be shared through electronic records is the Share2Care e-Xchange program, described in Box 8.2 (Fig. 8.4).

Box 8.2

Share2Care e-Xchange program (Cheshire and Merseyside, Lancashire and South Cumbria, United Kingdom).

The Share2Care e-Xchange Program aims to join up digital services across Cheshire and Merseyside, Lancashire and South Cumbria (UK) to improve communication between health and care organizations. Authorized healthcare professionals use the platform to view patient information held by different health and care organizations in the region. This allows the patient's clinical information to be available

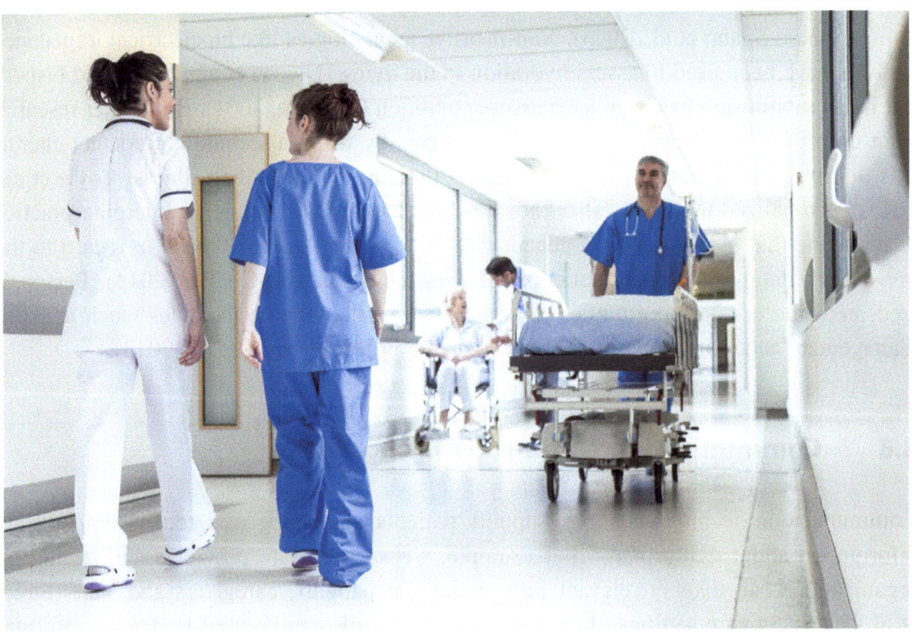

Fig. 8.4 *Credit* Spotmatik Ltd./Shutterstock

to the right professionals, in the right place, at the right time, so they can make a more informed clinical assessment and decisions.

The Electronic Palliative Care Coordination Systems (EPaCCS) sits within this program and aims to ensure that all involved healthcare professionals can access relevant information, including any changes to their preferences and wishes and personalized care plans.

8.9 Technology in Bereavement Support

Technologies can be used to support bereaved people in several different ways. In the digital age, there are an increasing number of online services to support bereaved people (e.g., governmental, health, educational, social media, conventional media, spiritual), which offer a different types of support for users (e.g., practical support, services, peer support, informational support, resources) (Beaunoyer et al., 2020). Options to deliver formal bereavement support (traditionally conducted face-to-face) could be expanded through telehealth (Stanley et al., 2024), online resources, virtual counselling sessions or online peer support (Coret and Martimianakis, 2023; Bassett, 2015). From a digital legacy perspective, technology could be purposively used to create and archive digital media (e.g., photos, videos, messages) to provide comfort to those experiencing grief and bereavement (Guenther et al., 2022). Digital legacy has added importance, as grief can be further complicated if bereaved people are unable to access digital media of the deceased person (e.g., because the lack passwords and permissions to access the media), which may have sentimental significance, such as photographs, videos, voice recordings and music playlists (Robinson and Pond, 2019; Wagner et al., 2020). AI technologies are increasingly used by bereaved persons to interact with digital avatars of the deceased (Stein et al., 2019; Stanley et al., 2024). For example, HereAfterAI (https://www.hereafter.ai) preserves memories of individuals by supporting the user to create a biography of their life, by answering questions from a virtual interviewer. Following the users' death, living friends and family talk to a virtual representation of the deceased, that responds to questions with the answers provided by the deceased person when they were alive (described in Box 8.3). Other examples include, StoryFile (https://storyfile.com), which allows a user to create a conversational video AI avatar that responds to spoken questions, meaning that a user talks to a video representation of the dead person. Also, AI companion apps like Replika (https://replika.com) and Nomi (https://nomi.ai) provides users with the opportunity to recreate the likeness of the deceased person, by shaping the appearance, personality and speech of the avatar (Fig. 8.5).

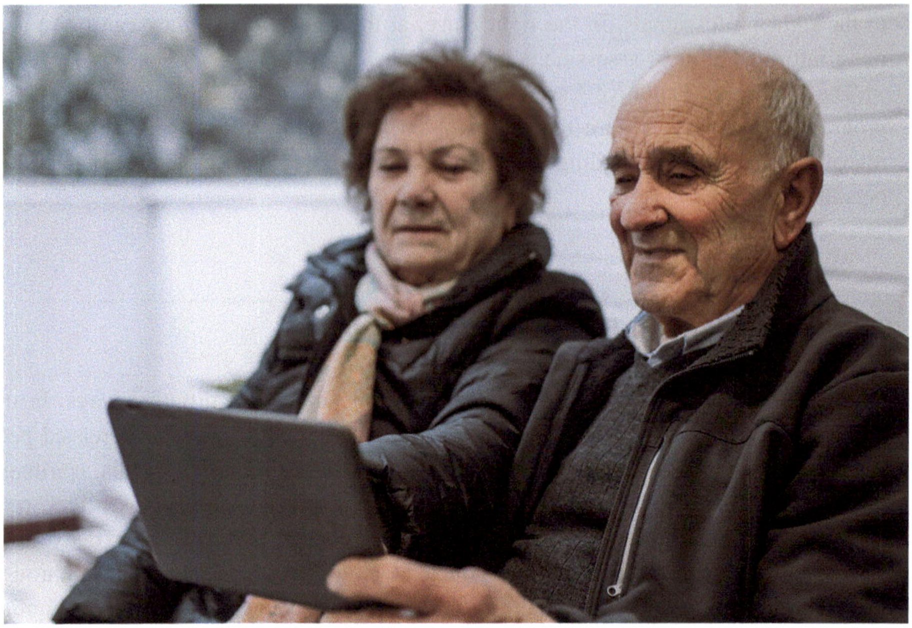

Fig. 8.5 *Credit* Carballo/Shutterstock

Box 8.3
HereAfterAI (https://www.hereafter.ai).

HereAfter AI is an app that uses AI to help people record and share their life stories, allowing loved ones to interact with these stories and memories in an interactive way after the person has died. The app aims to preserve and share memories and life stories in an interactive format, enabling users to connect with loved ones who have died by using their own voices to answer questions. The app uses a virtual interviewer to help users to audio record stories about their childhoods, relationships, experiences, and more. Authorised family members and friends can then ask questions to the app, which will access the recorded memories and respond in the person's voice, whilst also displaying photos.

8.10 Artificial Intelligence Applications to Support Care at the End-of-Life

Generative AI refers to deep-learning models that can generate high-quality text, images, and other content based on the data they were trained on (Fui-Hoon Nah et al., 2023). Generative AI uses algorithms, which are trained on large amounts of data, to determine patterns and create new content. As discussed in Sect. 8.9, generative AI has applications in palliative care, with companies using generative AI to create memorials to commemorate deceased (Wiederhold, 2024). For example, generative AI can be used to create messages, videos, or digital portraits to commemorate a person after death (Pataranutaporn et al., 2023). Generative AI can also be used to create interactive digital clones (avatars) of a deceased person by using AI tools for voice cloning (e.g., https://www.resemble.ai) face cloning (e.g., https://www.visionstory.ai) and text to speech generators (e.g., https://elevenlabs.io) (Wahba et al., 2024). VR and AR technologies can be used by living people to interact with digital clones, to ask questions, share memories and virtually attend social events (Chague and Charbonnier, 2015). These technologies, used in combination with voice cloning technologies, create opportunities for users to create interactive digital avatars, which have the characteristics of the deceased person. Generative AI applications like LiveMemory (https://www.myheritage.com/livememory) and Luma AI Dream Machine (https://lumalabs.ai/dream-machine), provides users with the ability convert still photos into an animated video, which could be used to bring memories of the deceased 'back to life' or reimagine the scene completely differently.

These generative AI tools offer new opportunities for bereaved people to remember the dead, and it also provides a new modality for the living to curate, and archive, their memories in a digital format. There is a lack of policy to guide practitioners, and the public, of how personal data (in the form of images and videos) should be accessed (and used) after death (Norris et al., 2022). This lack of policy creates challenges about ownership, access, consent and misuse of digital assets after death (Norris et al., 2022). Furthermore, there are several ethical and social challenges of using generative AI to alter or create memories. For example, editing images may lead to a loss of authenticity and a distorted reality, as it is possible that the use of generative AI to alter images could lead to replacement of genuine memories, leading to a loss of the true essence of past experiences. For further discussion about ethical issues relating to AI avatars and palliative care, please refer to Sect. 10.15. For further discussion about ethical issues relating to AI and AgeTech in general, please refer to Sect. 10.2.

8.11 Key Initiatives

There are many benefits of collaborative working to support person centered care at the end-of-life, and existing initiatives encourage this approach. The initiatives discussed below empower the patient to be central to their own care planning.

The Integrated Mersey Palliative Care Team (IMPaCT)
IMPaCT is a UK partnership between Marie Curie Hospice (Liverpool), Mersey Care NHS Foundation Trust, Liverpool University Hospitals NHS Foundation Trust and Woodlands Hospice. IMPacCT includes a telehealth service to provide support to people with a life limiting condition 24 h a day, 7 days a week. Healthcare professionals from local hospitals, hospices and communities are available to support health issues, maintaining quality of life and planning future care. Following contact with the patient, health records are updated and shared between local healthcare providers to offer a joined-up approach to palliative care.

Talk CPR (Live Now)
Talk CPR is an awareness campaign in association with 'Byw Nawr—Live Now' in Wales, UK (https://talkcpr.wales). The aim of this initiative is to encourage conversation about Cardiopulmonary Resuscitation (CPR) for people affected by life-limiting and palliative illnesses. This web-based resource, featuring written information and YouTube videos, provides information for both patients and healthcare professionals, encouraging discussions around Do not attempt Cardiopulmonary Resuscitation (DNACPR).

8.12 Find Out More

The Digital Preservation Coalition.

https://www.dpconline.org/digipres.

The Digital Legacy Association.

https://digitallegacyassociation.org.

Share2Care e-Xchange program.

https://www.share2care.nhs.uk/Home.

HereAfterAI.

(https://www.hereafter.ai).

The Integrated Mersey Palliative Care Team (IMPaCT).

https://www.merseycare.nhs.uk/our-services/liverpool/integrated-mersey-palliative-care-team-impact.

Talk CPR.

https://talkcpr.wales.

References

Adam, R., de Bruin, M., Burton, C. D., Bond, C. M., Clausen, M. G. & Murchie, P. 2018. What are the current challenges of managing cancer pain and could digital technologies help? *BMJ supportive & palliative care*, 8, 204–212.

Avati, A., Jung, K., Harman, S., Downing, L., Ng, A. & Shah, N. H. 2018. Improving palliative care with deep learning. *BMC Med Inform Decis Mak*, 18, 122.

Barbato, M. 2001. Bispectral index monitoring in unconscious palliative care patients. *Journal of Palliative Care*, 17, 102–108.

Bassett, D. J. 2015. Who wants to live forever? Living, dying and grieving in our digital society. *Social Sciences*, 4, 1127–1139.

Beaunoyer, E., Torres, L. H., Maessen, L. & Guitton, M. J. 2020. Grieving in the digital era: Mapping online support for grief and bereavement. *Patient Education and Counseling*, 103, 2515–2524.

Bellamy, C., Arnold, M., Gibbs, M., Nansen, B. & Kohn, T. Life beyond the timeline: creating and curating a digital legacy. meeting of Prato Community Informatics Research Network (CIRN), Prato, Italy, 2013.

Bernacki, R., Hutchings, M., Vick, J., Smith, G., Paladino, J., Lipsitz, S., Gawande, A. A. & Block, S. D. 2015. Development of the Serious Illness Care Program: a randomised controlled trial of a palliative care communication intervention. *BMJ open*, 5, e009032.

Brett, K. & Severn, M. 2023. Facial analysis technology for pain detection: a potentially useful tool for people living with dementia. *Canadian Journal of Health Technologies*, 3.

Bruehl, S., Apkarian, A. V., Ballantyne, J. C., Berger, A., Borsook, D., Chen, W. G., Farrar, J. T., Haythornthwaite, J. A., Horn, S. D. & Iadarola, M. J. 2013. Personalized medicine and opioid analgesic prescribing for chronic pain: opportunities and challenges. *The Journal of Pain*, 14, 103–113.

Ceci, L. 2022. TikTok: Number of global users 2020–2025. Statista. https://www.statista.com/statistics/1327116/number-of-global….

Chague, S. & Charbonnier, C. Digital cloning for an increased feeling of presence in collaborative virtual reality environments. International Conference on D Body Scanning Technologies, 2015.

Coret, M. & Martimianakis, M. A. 2023. Conceptualizations of "good death" and their relationship to technology: A scoping review and discourse analysis. *Health Science Reports*, 6, e1374.

Coyle, S., Chapman, E., Hughes, D. M., Baker, J., Slater, R., Davison, A. S., Norman, B. P., Roberts, I., Nwosu, A. C., Gallagher, J. A., Ranganath, L. R., Boyd, M. T., Mayland, C. R., Kell, D. B., Mason, S., Ellershaw, J. & Probert, C. 2025. Urinary metabolite model to predict the dying process in lung cancer patients. *Communications Medicine*, 5, 49.

Dash, J., Haller, D. M., Sommer, J. & Junod Perron, N. 2016. Use of email, cell phone and text message between patients and primary-care physicians: cross-sectional study in a French-speaking part of Switzerland. *BMC health services research*, 16, 1–7.

Doyle, A., Sharma, M. L., Gupta, M., Goebel, A. & Marley, K. 2022. Percutaneous cervical cordotomy for cancer-related pain: prospective multimodal outcomes evaluation. *BMJ Supportive & Palliative Care*, 12, e21–e27.

Durieux, B. N., Tarbi, E. C. & Lindvall, C. 2022. Opportunities for computational tools in palliative care: Supporting patient needs and lowering burden. SAGE Publications Sage UK: London, England.

Easwar, S., Alonzi, S., Hirsch, J., Mossman, B. & Hoerger, M. 2022. Palliative Care TikTok: Describing the Landscape and Explaining Social Media Engagement. *Journal of Palliative Medicine*, 26, 360–365.

Favela, J., Rodríguez, M., Preciado, A. & González, V. M. 2004. Integrating context-aware public displays into a mobile hospital information system. *IEEE transactions on information technology in Biomedicine*, 8, 279–286.

Fui-Hoon Nah, F., Zheng, R., Cai, J., Siau, K. & Chen, L. 2023. Generative AI and ChatGPT: Applications, challenges, and AI-human collaboration. Taylor & Francis.

Graham, F. & Clark, D. 2005. The syringe driver and the subcutaneous route in palliative care: the inventor, the history and the implications. *Journal of pain and symptom management*, 29, 32–40.

Guenther, M., Görlich, D., Bernhardt, F., Pogatzki-Zahn, E., Dasch, B., Krueger, J. & Lenz, P. 2022. Virtual reality reduces pain in palliative care–A feasibility trial. *BMC Palliative Care*, 21, 169.

HAMIDI, M., MAHENDRAN, P. & DENECKE, K. 2019. Towards a digital lean hospital: concept for a digital patient board and its integration with a hospital information system. *MEDINFO 2019: Health and Wellbeing e-Networks for All.* IOS Press.

Hua, Y., Wu, D., Gao, T., Liu, L., He, Y., Ding, Y., Rao, Q., Wu, Q. & Zhao, Z. 2023. Minimally invasive interventional therapy for pain. *Journal of Interventional Medicine*, 6, 64–68.

Jackson, S. E. & Chester, J. D. 2015. Personalised cancer medicine. *International journal of cancer*, 137, 262–266.

Malhotra, C., Shafiq, M. & Batcagan-Abueg, A. P. M. 2022. What is the evidence for efficacy of advance care planning in improving patient outcomes? A systematic review of randomised controlled trials. *BMJ open*, 12, e060201.

Marchal, F., Brunaud, L., Bazin, C., Boccacini, H., Henrot, P., Troufleau, P., Krakowski, I. & Regent, D. 2006. Radiofrequency ablation in palliative supportive care: early clinical experience. *Oncology reports*, 15, 495–499.

Norris, J. & Sofka, C. 2025. *Digital Death Report 2025—Digital Legacy Association* [Online]. Available: https://digitallegacyassociation.org/about/reports-2/ [Accessed].

Norris, J., Sofka, C. & Ging, T. 2022. *Why Digital Assets planning and Digital Legacy safeguarding should form a holistic approach to advance care planning* [Online]. Available: https://www.researchgate.net/publication/364209840_Why_Digital_Assets_planning_and_Digital_Legacy_safeguarding_should_form_a_holistic_approach_to_advance_care_planning [Accessed].

Norris, J. 2024. *P-138 Dying in today's digital world, societal and healthcare perspectives in 2024* [Online]. British Medical Journal Publishing Group. Available: https://spcare.bmj.com/content/14/Suppl_4/A62.1 [Accessed].

Nwosu, A. C., Mcglinchey, T., Sanders, J., Stanley, S., Palfrey, J., Lubbers, P., Chapman, L., Finucane, A. & Mason, S. 2022. Identification of digital health priorities for palliative care research: modified delphi study. *JMIR aging*, 5, e32075.

Nwosu, A. C., Stanley, S., Mayland, C. R., Mason, S., Mcdougall, A. & Ellershaw, J. E. 2024. Non-invasive technology to assess hydration status in advanced cancer to explore relationships between fluid status and symptoms: an observational study using bioelectrical impedance analysis. *BMC Palliative Care*, 23, 209.

Paolini, F., Ferini, G., Bonosi, L., Costanzo, R., Brunasso, L., Benigno, U. E., Porzio, M., Gerardi, R. M., Giammalva, G. R. & Umana, G. E. 2022. Spinal cord stimulation to treat unresponsive cancer pain: a possible solution in palliative oncological therapy. *Life*, 12, 554.

Pataranutaporn, P., Danry, V., Blanchard, L., Thakral, L., Ohsugi, N., Maes, P. & Sra, M. Living memories: AI-generated characters as digital mementos. Proceedings of the 28th International Conference on Intelligent User Interfaces, 2023. 889–901.

Petrova, M., Riley, J., Abel, J. & Barclay, S. 2018. Crash course in EPaCCS (Electronic Palliative Care Coordination Systems): 8 years of successes and failures in patient data sharing to learn from. *BMJ supportive & palliative care*, 8, 447–455.

Robinson, C. & Pond, R. 2019. Do online support groups for grief benefit the bereaved? Systematic review of the quantitative and qualitative literature. *Computers in Human Behavior*, 100, 48–59.

Sandic Spaho, R., Uhrenfeldt, L., Fotis, T. & Kymre, I. G. 2023. Wearable devices in palliative care for people 65 years and older: A scoping review. *Digital Health*, 9, 20552076231181212.

Simpson, K. H. 2011. Interventional techniques for pain management in palliative care. *Medicine*, 39, 645–647.

Stanley, S., Finucane, A., Thompson, A. & Nwosu, A. C. 2024. How can technology be used to support communication in palliative care beyond the covid-19 pandemic: a mixed-methods national survey of palliative care healthcare professionals. *BMC palliative care*, 23, 40.

Stanley, S., Higginbotham, K., Finucane, A. & Nwosu, A. C. 2023. A grounded theory study exploring palliative care healthcare professionals' experiences of managing digital legacy as part of advance care planning for people receiving palliative care. *Palliative Medicine*, 02692163231194198.

Stein, C. H., Hartl Majcher, J., Froemming, M. W., Greenberg, S. C., Benoit, M. F., Gonzales, S. M., Petrowski, C. E., Mattei, G. M. & Dulek, E. B. 2019. Community psychology, digital technology, and loss: Remembrance activities of young adults who have experienced the death of a close friend. *Journal of community & applied social psychology*, 29, 257–272.

Street, A. F., Swift, K., Annells, M., Woodruff, R., Gliddon, T., Oakley, A. & Ottman, G. 2007. Developing a web-based information resource for palliative care: an action-research inspired approach. *BMC Medical Informatics and Decision Making*, 7, 1–13.

Suhardjono, L. A. The Use of Digital Technologies in the Art World to Preserve Traumatic Cultural Legacies. E3S Web of Conferences, 2023. EDP Sciences, 02047.

Taubert, M., Watts, G., Boland, J. & Radbruch, L. 2014. Palliative social media. *BMJ Supportive & Palliative Care*, 4, 13–18.

The Digital Legacy Association. 2024. *The Digital Legacy Association* [Online]. The website of the Digital Legacy Association. Available: https://digitallegacyassociation.org/ [Accessed 2025].

Wagner, B., Rosenberg, N., Hofmann, L. & Maass, U. 2020. Web-based bereavement care: a systematic review and meta-analysis. *Frontiers in psychiatry*, 11, 537629.

Wahba, K. A., Ahmed, K. A., Kamel, M. R., Fathy, M., Abdelfatah, P. K. H. & Hatem, S. Creating a Digital Human Twin: Cloning Voice, Face, and Attitude. 2024 International Mobile, Intelligent, and Ubiquitous Computing Conference (MIUCC), 2024. IEEE, 199–205.

Wiederhold, B. K. 2024. Monuments and Memorials: A Role for Artificial Intelligence in the Grieving Process. Mary Ann Liebert, Inc., publishers 140 Huguenot Street, 3rd Floor New ….

9 Conducting AgeTech Research in Palliative Care

9.1 The Challenge

The previous chapters have highlighted several important interconnected themes, which describe how AgeTech can support delivery of palliative care. In describing these themes, we have provided an overview of how AgeTech technologies can be used to address specific palliative care needs of older people. We have also described the practical considerations (e.g., opportunities and challenges) of using AgeTech in clinical practice. Research is essential to identify how these technologies can be used well in practice and overcome the barriers of its implementation. However, there are many factors which create challenges for palliative care research, which reduces the potential to improve care through evidence-based approaches. There are several challenges affecting research of palliative care AgeTech. Broadly, these may include issues with funding, research methodology, ethics, consent, research governance, cost effectiveness and impact. We will explore these aspects in greater detail below (Fig. 9.1).

9.2 Funding Challenges

There is little public funding for palliative care research. Consequently, palliative care researchers need to compete on an 'open market' against other researchers within (and outside) of their discipline, to secure funding to conduct palliative care research. In the UK, less than 0.3% of the £500 million spent on cancer research is allocated to palliative care; furthermore, funding for non-cancer conditions is likely to be less (NCRI cancer database 2016—Higginson 2016). This lack of funding limits the opportunities for palliative care research to be conducted. This lack of research means that the evidence needed to improve palliative care (including AgeTech) is not being generated.

A. C. Nwosu et al., *Technologies in Palliative Care for Older People*, Synthesis Lectures on Technology and Health, https://doi.org/10.1007/978-3-032-04277-4_9

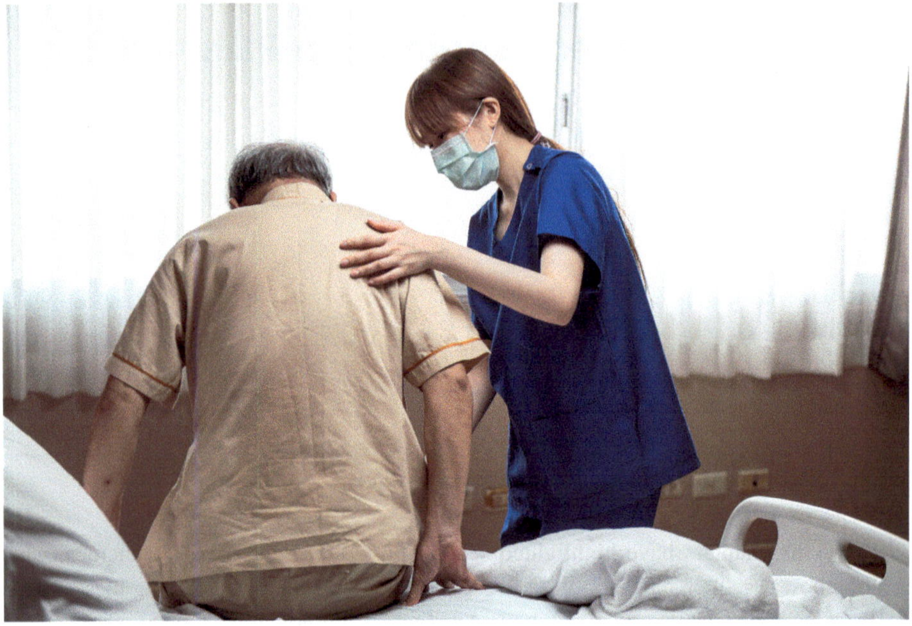

Fig. 9.1 *Credit* Cat Box/Shutterstock

9.3 Methodological Challenges

Palliative care has developed outside of traditional medical and higher education institutions, restricting the academic development of the specialty (Kaasa and Radbruch, 2008). Currently, there are limitations to the evidence base of palliative medicine, as most published studies are small and lack internationally agreed core-outcome measures, which means it is difficult to compare findings between research investigators (Higginson, 2016).

Research involving dying people is methodologically and ethically challenging, as they often have significant symptomatic burden (such as pain, fatigue and psychological distress) (Addington-Hall et al., 2007). Researchers may struggle to engage and recruit participants due to concerns about their ability to comply with assessments and provide consent (Kaasa and Radbruch, 2008). These problems may be further exacerbated by 'gatekeeping' behavior of healthcare staff and academics, who may limit opportunities for people with palliative care needs to participate in research, due to concerns that research involvement will cause distress (Kars et al., 2016). However, evidence demonstrates that people with serious illness want to be involved in palliative care research (White and Hardy, 2010). Therefore, limiting opportunities for people with palliative care needs to participate in research reduces their autonomy, and limits the ability to generate the research needed to inform clinical practice (Henderson et al., 2005; Payne et al.,

2013; Nwosu et al., 2013). Consequently, low levels of recruitment, small sample sizes and high attrition rates often have a negative impact on the methodological quality of research (Nwosu, 2012).

Research in AgeTech is further challenging due to the speed of digital health innovation, and a lack of researchers with the methodogical expertise this is required to evaluate these innovations. For example, in 2022 the artificial intelligence driven chatbot 'ChatGPT' was launched within seven years of the creation of OpenAI, which is much shorter than the usual 17 years for translational research to influence clinical practice (Morris et al., 2011).

9.4 Ethical Issues in AgeTech Research

Several ethical issues create challenges with conducting palliative care research. These include the following:

Informed Consent and autonomy: Older people with palliative care needs may find it challenging to consent for research due to factors such as cognitive impairment, pain, and emotional distress. Evidence demonstrates that people with palliative care needs generally want to participate in research, therefore it is important that researchers design studies to address the needs of those receiving palliative care (e.g., using methods to enable participants to consent to palliative (and end-of-life) care research 'in advance' of their expected deterioration) (Rees and Hardy, 2003; Coyle et al., 2016).

Ensuring benefit and avoiding harm: It is important that researchers maximize benefits (beneficence) and minimize harm (nonmaleficence) to participants of palliative care research. People with palliative care needs may have significant problems with their physical and mental health, which may make them vulnerable to harm. Consequently, it is important that AgeTech research is carefully designed for the needs of users, so they receive potential benefits of these interventions without experiencing unanticipated harm. For example, VR is a low-risk intervention, but it could potentially cause harm to frail participants who may experience discomfort from ill-fitting straps and bulky systems, with risks of cross-infection between patients if appropriate procedures are not followed (Nwosu et al., 2024). Researchers should consider the possibility of wider unintentional 'harms' which may be associated with AgeTech research, for example the potential for grief, bereavement and attachment issues in studies using technologies to recreate the dead as digital avatars. Therefore, it is important to carefully evaluate the risks and potential benefits of AgeTech interventions specific to the needs of the older people with palliative care needs.

End-of-Life care and decision making: Palliative care research may involve sensitive topics related to end-of-life care and decision making, which may include areas such as symptom management, dying care, bereavement, advance care planning and euthanasia. AgeTech researchers should be aware of these issues and design projects carefully to ensure that participant's end-of-life care is supported, and researched, acknowledging the preferences of participants. Researchers should consider how AgeTech adds new dimensions to palliative care issues and to identify the safeguards required to ensure that care is not compromised (for example, AI algorithms which provide inaccurate survival predictions may negatively influence healthcare practitioners decision making).

Confidentiality and Privacy: AgeTech researchers need to implement appropriate measures to safeguard data and ensure confidentiality and privacy of palliative care participants. This is increasingly important due to the increased use of health data, and technologies which analyze this data, which may create challenges of identifying those responsible for protecting the rights of users (e.g., what are the roles and responsibilities of healthcare professionals, organizations and health tech companies when managing health (and personal) data of its users?).

Equality and equity: Researchers should consider the factors which affect the equality in AgeTech use. Issues such as cost, cultural issues (e.g., language), design, bias and geography may reduce the transferability of AgeTech to different groups, potentially creating inequity in healthcare delivery. For example, technologies using artificial intelligence powered algorithms, may not represent certain groups (e.g., minorities) if the data of these groups was not used in the development of the algorithms (Ashwini, 2024).

9.5 Overcoming the Challenges in Palliative Care AgeTech Research

We have provided an overview of the infrastructural, methodological and ethical issues, which researchers should consider when conducting AgeTech research for older people with palliative care needs. The above challenges highlight the importance of ensuring AgeTech research in palliative care is conducted with a team who have expertise and knowledge of the methodological challenges for AgeTech research and how to overcome these challenges. Teams should be multidisciplinary, reflecting the skills that are necessary for the work. This may include research methodologists, statisticians, computer scientists, ethicists, engineers, designers, and healthcare professionals. AgeTech research offers an exciting opportunity to explore how new technologies can be used to support care; however, it is necessary that important methodological issues are addressed.

9.6 Find Out More

European Association for Palliative Care (EAPC) blog—Artificial Intelligence has no role in palliative care…or does it?
https://eapcnet.wordpress.com/2023/03/07/artificial-intelligence-has-no-role-in-palliative-care-or-does-it/.

Futurism in Palliative: An overview of the Palliative Care, Architecture and Design Symposium (PADS 2018).

https://eapcnet.wordpress.com/2019/02/25/futurism-in-palliative-an-overview-of-the-palliative-care-architecture-and-design-symposium-pads-2018/.

Identification of Digital Health Priorities for Palliative Care Research: Modified Delphi Study.

https://aging.jmir.org/2022/1/e32075/.

References

Addington-Hall, J. M., Bruera, E., Higginson, I. J. & Payne, S. 2007. *Research methods in palliative care*, OUP Oxford.

Ashwini, K. 2024. Contemporary forms of racism, racial discrimination, xenophobia and related intolerance: report of the Special Rapporteur on Contemporary Forms of Racism, Racial Discrimination, Xenophobia and Related Intolerance, Ashwini KP.

Coyle, S., Scott, A., Nwosu, A. C., Latten, R., Wilson, J., Mayland, C. R., Mason, S., Probert, C. & Ellershaw, J. 2016. Collecting biological material from palliative care patients in the last weeks of life: a feasibility study. *BMJ Open,* 6, e011763.

Henderson, M., Addington-Hall, J. M. & Hotopf, M. 2005. The willingness of palliative care patients to participate in research. *J Pain Symptom Manage,* 29, 116–8.

Higginson, I. J. 2016. Research challenges in palliative and end of life care. *BMJ Supportive & Palliative Care,* 6, 2–4.

Kaasa, S. & Radbruch, L. 2008. Palliative care research--priorities and the way forward. *Eur J Cancer,* 44, 1175–9.

Kars, M. C., van Thiel, G. J., van der Graaf, R., Moors, M., de Graeff, A. & van Delden, J. J. 2016. A systematic review of reasons for gatekeeping in palliative care research. *Palliative medicine,* 30, 533–548.

Morris, Z. S., Wooding, S. & Grant, J. 2011. The answer is 17 years, what is the question: understanding time lags in translational research. *Journal of the royal society of medicine,* 104, 510–520.

Nwosu, A. C., Mills, M., Roughneen, S., Stanley, S., Chapman, L. & Mason, S. R. 2024. Virtual reality in specialist palliative care: a feasibility study to enable clinical practice adoption. *BMJ supportive & palliative care,* 14, 47–51.

Nwosu, A. C., Mayland, C. R., Mason, S., Varro, A. & Ellershaw, J. E. 2013. Patients want to be involved in end-of-life care research. *BMJ Supportive & Palliative Care.*

Nwosu, A. C. 2012. Integrated clinical academic training: an exciting new dawn for academic palliative medicine. *J Palliat Med,* 15**,** 507–8.

Payne, S., Preston, N., Turner, M. & Rolls, L. 2013. Research in palliative care—can hospices afford to not be involved?: International Observatory on End of Life Care, University of Lancaster.

Rees, E. & Hardy, J. 2003. Novel consent process for research in dying patients unable to give consent. *BMJ,* 327**,** 198.

White, C. & Hardy, J. 2010. What do palliative care patients and their relatives think about research in palliative care?-a systematic review. *Support Care Cancer,* 18**,** 905–11.

10 Emerging Issues and Future Directions

The authors have worked on various sections and contributed comments and shared feedback to prepare this book. We have identified several unifying emerging themes for further discussion of their importance for future direction for practice, policy and research in AgeTech for older people with palliative care needs. We received useful feedback from reviewers of an early draft of the manuscript, which highlighted key ideas and themes relating to the opportunities or challenges of using AgeTech in 'real world' palliative care environments. Our discussion of 'real world' environments highlights important clinical practice issues regarding AgeTech in palliative care, such as consent, governance, data management issues, ethical challenges and equity. This final chapter summarizes the main areas of our discussion and reflects on future areas of focus, for practitioners, researchers, policy makers and society (Fig. 10.1).

10.1 Limitations of This Book

We acknowledge there are limitations with this book which may reduce the transferability of the findings to certain audiences. Firstly, this book is first written in English, with the four authors residing in the United Kingdom; therefore, we acknowledge the Western geographical and cultural focus of the narrative. We acknowledge that many of the examples of innovation in this book describes European, North American and Australian developments and perspectives, meaning that AgeTech developments in other countries (e.g., Asia, African and South America) may not be fully explored. One explanation for the Western focus is that AgeTech innovations are generally prevalent in areas experiencing aging populations, meaning that AgeTech innovations are generally obserevd

A. C. Nwosu et al., *Technologies in Palliative Care for Older People*, Synthesis Lectures on Technology and Health, https://doi.org/10.1007/978-3-032-04277-4_10

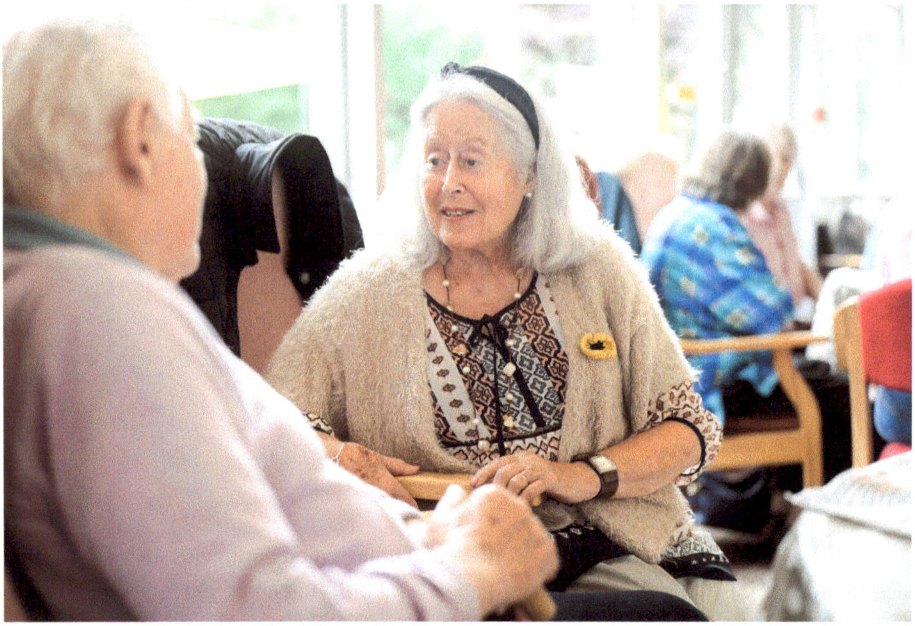

Fig. 10.1 *Credit* Bramley Elderly action/aging better

in aging Western populations. We acknowledge that population aging is important in Asian countries (e.g., Japan, China and South Korea); however, we were unable access some information due to the language barrier. Previous studies demonstrate the emerging importance of palliative care digital health in Asia Pacific, Australasia and Africa. Australian palliative care providers report digital health priorities, with providers promoting innovations in health record management, telehealth, and personal health tracking (Mills et al., 2021a). Digital health priorities are likely to differ between countries due to geopolitical and socioeconomic drivers (Nwosu et al., 2022). For example, in Sub-Saharan African, digital health is not as established when compared to other developed regions (Allsop et al., 2018). Consequently, Sub-Saharan African stakeholders describe digital health as part of a wider vision in this region, to potentially improve data management and to support the development of healthcare services (Nkhoma et al., 2021; Ngoma et al., 2021). Palliative care is a growing discipline in the Asia Pacific region and there is limited research describing digital health priorities, although there is acknowledgement that digital health can play an important role in supporting staff and student education and training (Mills et al., 2021b).

The authors of this book acknowledge that their interest in digital health may promote a positive presentation of AgeTech in this synthesis. We acknowledge that our academic interest of the potential benefits of AgeTech has prompted the development of this book, and that it possible that the personas (and AgeTech examples) in this book present an idealized view of AgeTech in palliative care. It is evident that many factors are important in the delivery of person-centered palliative care, supported by AgeTech, and we appreciate that there are likely to be many contributing factors (important for real-world success), which have not been covered in this book. We purposely constructed personas around specific areas (such as communication, psychosocial care and end-of-life care) to help the reader to understand the potential, case-specific, benefits of AgeTech; however, we acknowledge this makes it challenging to describe how AgeTech addresses the needs of people transitioning between phases of illness. The physical and psychosocial needs of an AgeTech user will change as the user becomes increasingly weaker and requires more assistance. Unless carefully designed (and implemented), AgeTech may lack effectiveness in these transition points of illness, as a user moves from independence, to dependence, dying and then death. Consequently, the reader should acknowledge that the AgeTech presented in each persona is illustrative, and careful consideration is required to determine the real-world applicability across the changing course of illness in a person's life. It is also possible that digital health bias extends to researchers in the field of AgeTech, due to their interest in new technologies, with research participants more likely to identify as those with interest in digital technologies.

A consequence of focusing on AgeTech interventions, with individuals who are interested in digital technologies, is the risk of exclusion of those who are unable, or do not wish, to use AgeTech. This increases the risk of bias (where AgeTech tools are not developed for certain individuals due to lack of data, design and focus) and the potential that certain individuals will not be represented by these technologies (e.g., people with disabilities). It is challenging to provide patient and caregiver perspective of palliative care AgeTech, as this has not yet been fully explored in literature. Currently, most AgeTech research focuses on healthcare professionals' perspectives; therefore, future work to gain perspectives of the public, about palliative care AgeTech, is urgently required.

10.2 Ethical Considerations for Use of AgeTech in Palliative Care

It is important to consider ethical issues which are associated with AgeTech in palliative care. AgeTech can potentially offer benefits and harm for individuals and groups, depending on the circumstances of its use. Ethical theories represent different viewpoints, priorities and rules about decision-making; therefore, these theories are useful to provide a framework for using AgeTech in palliative care. Many ethical models exist, but the four principles are well known and commonly used in medical ethics. The four principles are a set of goals, to guide practice (and further understand the different ethical theories). The four ethical principles (beneficence, non-maleficence, autonomy and justice) were proposed by Beauchamp and Childress (Beauchamp and Childress, 1994), to help people to analyze bioethical dilemmas (Gillon, 1994, Gillon, 2015).

Beneficence: The requirement to act in the person's best interest. Practitioners should act in the person's best interests and take positive steps to promote the well-being of individuals. For example, practitioners should consider whether AgeTech is beneficial for the user. This may be relevant in situations where AgeTech has wider benefits for stakeholders but the benefits to individual users are uncertain.

Non-Maleficence (Do no harm): This principle requires practitioners to avoid actions that could cause unnecessary harm or suffering to patients. Using a 'do no harm' focus, practitioners would avoid AgeTech applications which harm individuals (e.g., physical, social, psychological, financial). For example, practitioners may view the potential risk of a user experiencing distress from viewing an AI avatar of a deceased relative as reason to not use this technology; however, other users may find this use of AgeTech beneficial.

Autonomy: This principle requires practitioners to respect the individuals' right to make their own decisions. With this approach, it is ethically important that practitioners ensure an individual has the right to independently make decisions about an intervention, which often requires the person to have the opportunity to consider the risks and benefits of the proposed action. An AgeTech example includes the critical ethical issue of obtaining consent to use historical patient data (such as data on electronic databases) for analysis different from the purpose for which the data was originally collected.

Justice: This principle emphasizes individual human rights and freedoms, the rule of law, and the values of fairness and justice. Guided by the principle of justice, practitioners should ensure that resources are distributed fairly, and individuals should have fair access. There is a risk of inequity (and hence, lack of justice) among older people accessing AgeTech, due to high costs associated with its development, maintenance and use. Inequality of access to AgeTech is counter to ethical principle of justice.

The four ethical principles are commonly used as a basis for ethical theories. Ethical theories are philosophical attempts to explain human morality. Four traditional ethical theories have been proposed by philosophers to guide ethical decision making, by defining what constitutes 'right' and 'wrong' actions in different situations. The four traditional ethical theories are known as consequentialism, deontology, virtue and rights-based (Chonko, 2012).

Consequentialism focuses on the outcomes of medical decisions and is often described by the phrase: 'the ends justify the means'. In consequentialism, an action is deemed ethical if the achieved outcome is deemed to be favorable, irrespective of the methods used to achieve this. For example, a practitioner may prioritize AgeTech interventions that benefit the greatest number of people, even if individual sacrifices are necessary (e.g., AI analytics, when applied to Electronic Patient Record (EPR) data, is effective for informing population-based decision-making and generating useful insights for large groups. However, this process uses the data of individuals who may not personally receive any direct benefit from the analysis).

Deontology emphasizes the importance of respecting moral rules and duties in practice. A deontological perspective requires healthcare practitioners to prioritize the autonomy of individuals, confidentiality, and informed consent as a priority, over the potential benefits of an intervention. For example, the practitioners using an algorithm to identify ways to generate funds for a healthcare service, need to ensure patient data was not unlawfully accessed or sold to third-parties.

Virtue Ethics focuses on the character of practitioners and their intent to act with compassion, integrity, and competence. For example, a virtuous practitioner would be guided by 'virtuous principles' to provide the best care for their patients and determine whether the use (or non-use) of AgeTech is consistent with their aim to act in the person's best interests.

Rights-Based Ethics focuses on respecting and upholding the rights of individuals, such as the right to life, privacy, and access to healthcare. For example, ensuring that individuals have the right to make informed decisions about whether they wish to use AgeTech and that the technology does not violate their right to privacy.

While medical ethical theories and the four principles provide a useful framework for guiding practitioners' decision-making, they can also create challenges due to conflicts between principles or ambiguous situations that lack clear resolutions (Baldassarre et al., 2023). Additionally, these ethical models largely stem from a Western perspective and may not fully account for the diverse cultural beliefs and values that shape ethical decision-making in different societies (Varkey, 2021). As cultures evolve, new societal norms, practices, and beliefs emerge, making traditional ethical models more difficult to apply universally. This challenge is particularly relevant with the advancement of technologies such as AI, which are reshaping cultural norms around the role of technology in human relationships (Floridi, 2023). The integration of AI into healthcare and other fields raises new ethical questions that may not be easily addressed by traditional ethical frameworks. For example, it is important to address specific issues such as accountability (who is responsible for AI systems if there is a problem?), clinical autonomy (what procedures should be followed when human practitioners disagree with AI informed recommendations?) trust (how can we trust that the AI models are efficacious and effective?) and governance (what regulatory systems are in place to ensure that AI is used safely and effectively?).

10.3 Accountability and Trust in Artificial Intelligence

Future developments in AI-focused AgeTech should be designed to limit potential harm which may result from inappropriate use of AI in palliative care. In this book we highlight some issues associated with algorithms, and other AI methods, providing treatment recommendations, which are developed without sufficient data about the patient cohort. There is potential that AI-focused methods may lack the ability to accurately inform palliative care treatment decisions, if the algorithms were not developed to adequately represent the specific attributes, and evolving needs, of older people with palliative care needs (Floridi, 2023). Problems with the accuracy of these models may create challenges about trust in the outcomes, and questions of accountability for harms (or other problems), which result from negative issues arising from AI in palliative care (Nwosu et al., 2018, 2022). Future policy and practice must ensure that algorithmic systems are safe and accountable. This requires transparency about how these systems generate recommendations, and clear identification of who is responsible for the resulting decisions and their consequences (Bajwa et al., 2021).

10.4 Palliative Care Needs of Older People, the Promise and Pitfalls of AgeTech

Global palliative care needs are increasing due to several socioeconomic factors, such as population aging and the increasing burden of non-cancer conditions (Etkind et al., 2017; Sleeman et al., 2019); therefore, it is important to explore opportunities to ensure that populations have adequate access to palliative care services (Bone et al., 2017). Digital health innovation in AgeTech offers potential to transform health and social care, and provide opportunities for citizens to manage their own health (Topol, 2019; Department of Health Social Care, 2018; Haghi et al., 2017). In this book we have covered several exciting scenarios where AgeTech can potentially support the palliative care needs of older people. Examples of the usefulness of AgeTech included themes in communication, long-term conditions, psychosocial care, coordination of care and end-of life-care. Furthermore, it is important to consider the general limitations of AgeTech in palliative care (e.g., expense, efficacy, efficiency interoperability issues, data privacy and security concerns and equality of access).

10.5 The COVID-19 Pandemic and Palliative Care AgeTech

This book was published after the end of the worldwide novel coronavirus (COVID-19) pandemic (Wise, 2023) but it is important to acknowledge that the pandemic accelerated the integration of AgeTech in palliative care practice (Stanley et al., 2024). Many of the future directions for AgeTech in palliative care are influenced by the technological shift that occurred in palliative care practice during the pandemic. The COVID-19 pandemic caused many palliative care services to rapidly implement technological solutions to reduce face-to-face human contact to limit virus transmission (Wherton et al., 2020). For example, telehealth was commonly used during the pandemic, with many palliative care services using this to provide remote clinical support (Calton et al., 2020, Grewal et al., 2020, Ritchey et al., 2020, Bettini, 2020, Chávarri-Guerra et al., 2020, Mackey et al., 2020, Harris et al., 2021, Flores et al., 2020, Lu et al., 2020, Sansom-Daly and Bradford, 2020, Samara et al., 2021, Chua et al., 2020, Lally et al., 2021), to communicate (Crosby et al., 2021) and for education (Lal et al., 2020). Technologies were used to maintain connection, and to develop communities of palliative care practice (Abel and Taubert, 2020) (Mills et al., 2020, Norris, 2020). VR was used to provide psychological care and symptom management (Niki et al., 2020; Taylor et al., 2021; Wang et al., 2020). In general, the findings of these studies describe potential benefits of digital health; however, the rapid implementation of these technologies has created several challenges (e.g., technical issues, data security and wellbeing considerations) which, require further evaluation (Crosby et al., 2021).

The impact of COVID-19 in increasing technology use in palliative care practice is likely to remain, partly due to newly developed innovations in care and education (Stanley et al., 2024), increasing awareness of end of life care needs (Norris and Sofka, 2025), and the increasing global need for palliative care (Sleeman et al., 2019).

10.6 Research Methodology in Palliative Care AgeTech Studies

Future research can use new AI analysis methods to evaluate care in real time, (Carbonell et al., 1983), which can support quality improvement in clinical practice (Greene et al., 2014; The Health Foundation, 2014). For example, Machine Learning techniques can be used to predict health outcomes of people as they age, in real-time, with existing information from the medical record (Esteva et al., 2017). Future AI applications may involve prognostic estimates (Yu et al., 2016), to provide treatment and therapy recommendations, and to support personalized treatment decisions based on an individual's characteristics, genetics and data (Chen et al., 2009). Despite its promise, the full potential of AI has not yet been fully realized in palliative care research, due to a lack of understanding of the methods, governance issues (e.g., related to data access and storage) and ethical issues. Further research, involving quantitative and qualitative longitudinal studies are needed to determine the efficacy, and effectiveness of AgeTech interventions. On a societal perspective, it is important to determine how to best use public resources to ensure AgeTech meaningfully supports the palliative care needs of older people (Nwosu, 2023; Finucane et al., 2020). It is important that future research involves an appropriately skilled group, with expertise in data science methods, palliative care and translational science, to ensure that the outcome of the research informs meaningful, real-world, use (Nwosu et al., 2022). As highlighted throughout this book, it is crucial that research studies focus on how AgeTech can meaningfully improve palliative care in real-world scenarios. This creates methodological and ethical considerations for future research, which uses novel data analysis methods. For example, rather than waiting for the end of a study to evaluate the benefit of an intervention, it may be possible to use AI methods to determine the effect of an AgeTech intervention at any time point of a prospective study, and then compare real-time data with matched data (i.e., of a similar population), to determine real-world outcomes. This presents opportunities and challenges of how to appropriately use AI in clinical research, to inform clinical care (Collins, 2016).

10.7 Communication in the Future

Technology's role in enhancing verbal and nonverbal communication is significant and will become increasingly vital to society. Furthermore, importance of both medicalized and non-medicalized technology in supporting healthcare professionals and aiding the decision-making process will also continue to grow. For example, some healthcare insurance providers are rewarding their clients to stay active and recording exercise with wearable devices (e.g., doing more than 5000 steps per day) (Coughlan, 2021). The evolving accuracy of these technologies, combined with the use of reliable biomarkers, will fundamentally change how we approach diagnosis, drug delivery, and patient management (Fig. 10.2).

It is likely that AgeTech will continue to provide different options for older people to communicate with healthcare providers (Stanley et al., 2024; Lally et al., 2021; Calton et al., 2020). Further developments in the use of virtual wards, telehealth, apps, social media, virtual reality, the internet and connected IoT devices, are likely to provide several opportunities to enable patients (and their caregivers) to access information and communicate with healthcare professionals (Jung, 2017, Stanley et al., 2024, Nwosu, 2023).

10.8 Physical Health in the Future

AgeTech has the potential to support the physical health of older people in several ways, which could support palliative care needs for this group. Research and policy work should consider the potential impact, and usefulness, of AgeTech for the following areas.

Enhanced Healthy Aging: AgeTech can be used to support older adults to lead healthier lives, with physical activity monitoring tools that can keep people active and engaged. At home, smart monitoring technologies, such as monitoring activities of daily living and

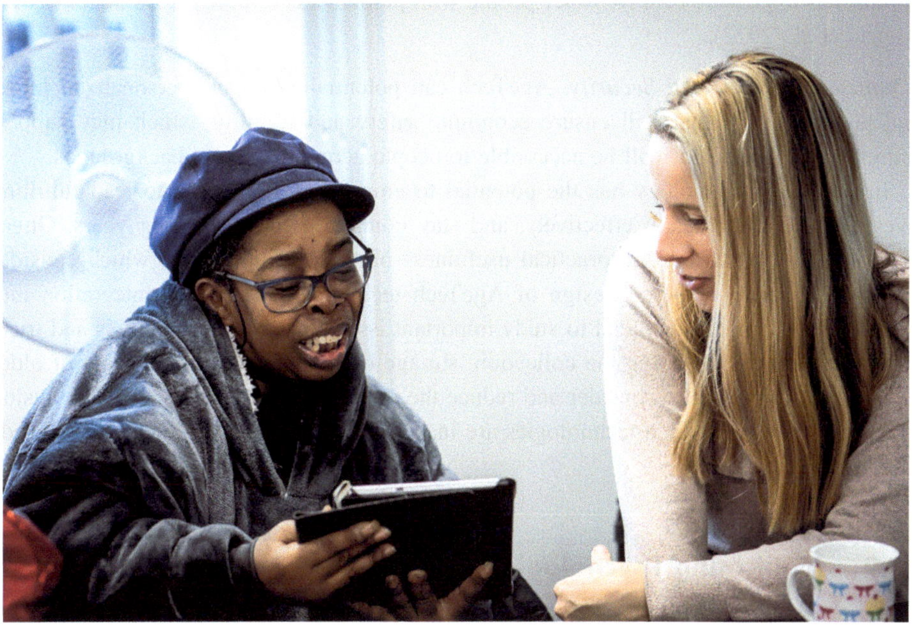

Fig. 10.2 *Credit* aging better

promoting safety (e.g., falls detection), offer opportunities to further support independent living.

Early Detection and Disease Management: AgeTech innovation in AI and digital biomarkers can potentially aid early disease detection. For example, wearable devices will track health status and connect with healthcare professionals remotely, with telemedicine facilitating personalized disease management at home.

Addressing Sensory Decline and Cognitive Functioning: Assistive technologies (e.g., robotics) have potential to further help compensate for sensory, and physical, decline. Furthermore, individuals can use AgeTech innovations to stabilize or improve their cognitive function.

Social Connection and Mental Well-being: Older adults can use digital platforms, and devices, to connect with their friends, family and community, potentially reducing social isolation. Researchers and policy makers should consider the importance of role of design, planning and architecture in incorporating AgeTech into compassionate communities, where technologies are used as a tool to improve social cohesion, compassion and palliative care. Technology-enabled care will likely increase in home and community environments, which improves opportunities for policymakers to use AgeTech in smart homes (Liu et al., 2016), and to support development of smart city, compassionate community approaches to provide care for older people with palliative care needs (Cook et al., 2018; Ahmad et al., 2022).

Financial Freedom and Security: AgeTech can potentially support personalized financial planning tools that will ensure economic safety and stability, which may support retirement planning that will be accessible to people across economic backgrounds.

In summary, technology has the potential to empower older adults to lead fulfilling lives, manage their health effectively, and stay connected in the coming years. Ongoing efforts are exploring the practical usefulness of these technologies, which consider appropriate human-centered design of AgeTech technologies and their integration into healthcare systems. It is crucial to study important issues of governance, ethics and trust, especially when considering the collection, storage of analysis of personal data of older people. It is important to consider and reduce the risk of harm, bias, and social exclusion that occurs when AgeTech technologies are inaccessible or unrepresentative of the needs of specific groups.

10.9 Monitoring Psychological Needs in the Future

Continued integration of technology in palliative care is enabling psychosocial care needs to be addressed in a more accessible and convenient way through telehealth, remote counselling and interactive therapeutic interventions. There is potential to improve monitoring of symptoms related to anxiety and depression to ensure care is delivered in a timely manner. For example, existing technologies could be further incorporated into practice to enable remote monitoring of anxiety related symptoms (Gomes et al., 2023). Wearable sensors are a widely available and often acceptable way of collecting data, which can be used for machine learning algorithms. Data linked to physiological changes (e.g., heart rate) and behavioural patterns (e.g., social interaction) can be monitored discreetly and conveniently. Remote monitoring of these symptoms could allow healthcare professionals to track psychological symptoms related to depression and anxiety, therefore helping to inform the need for psychological interventions in real time.

On a population level, use of wearable technologies to monitor psychological symptoms could provide greater insight into provision needs of the population, leading to more streamlined services to suit the needs of that population. However, considerations should be given to management and sharing of data to ensure that confidentiality is not at risk of being breeched.

10.10 Social Support in the Future

Rapid developments in the use of virtual reality (VR) and augmented reality (AR) have the potential to evolve and create highly immersive social spaces. The use of these technologies may offer opportunities for people to gather in a virtual community for support groups, therapy sessions, or to socialize; offering a sense of connection regardless of physical location. The development of 'virtual communities' may offer connectivity worldwide and could be user-generated. The use of virtual communities may potentially provide spaces for wellbeing activities, mental health support, and peer support. These spaces could incorporate virtual meditation sessions, yoga classes, therapy groups, and other activities aimed at promoting wellbeing and resilience.

10.11 Care Coordination in the Future

Technological advances in palliative care offer great opportunities to coordinate palliative care for older people. There are opportunities to better incorporate currently used technologies, in addition to using advances in AI, and other novel data analytics technologies, to improve care. For example, population level initiatives can aim to improve care coordination by increasing the coverage, and efficiency, of electronic care coordination systems. Improving the mechanisms of capture, use, and sharing digital health data can potentially improve care for service users, by enabling data to be meaningfully used. AI-driven analysis of EPR data has the potential to support large scale analysis, to rapidly provide data to inform clinical decisions about the palliative care needs of a population in a care setting or geographic area. For example, AI analysis of EPR data may be used to identify people with specific palliative care needs, to predict response to treatments, to predict survival and suggest population-level recommendations.

10.12 The Future of Creating Memories

Lifelogging devices, which records audio and visual data from a person's life, could become the future of memory making and curation. These devices have the potential to be developed in many ways, from wearables to companion robots. The future of memory curation could begin from birth and continue to death. Imagine that the teddy bear in the picture below (Fig. 10.3) was gifted to this child at birth. The bear could log memories and milestones throughout the owner's life. Devices could offer total recall to enable the user to review significant life events at their own will. Throughout life the owner could choose to carefully manage the memory bank contained in the device. Upon death, the owner could choose a recipient who would receive the device and access the memories

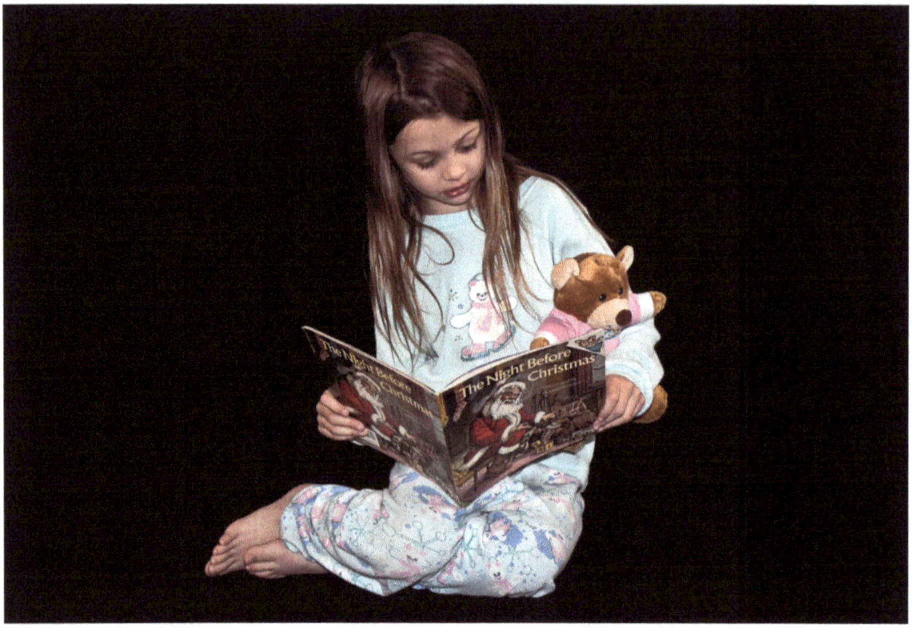

Fig. 10.3 *Credit* Jenn Durfey/Flickr

contained within it. However, there are ethical issues involving these developments which need to be considered, particularly around data privacy and sharing.

10.13 The Future of Digital Legacy Leadership: The Digital Legacy Association

Leadership is essential to ensure adequate policy and practice in the supporting people (and society) to manage digital assets, according to their wishes and preferences, ahead of their death (Nowaczyk-Basińska, 2025). Leadership in the field of digital legacy is provided by individuals (such as Professor Sofka (2012) and Dr. Kasket (2019)), and organizations like the Digital Legacy Association (2024). The Digital Legacy Association is a professional body with the strategic aim of raising public awareness in areas relating to digital assets planning and digital legacy safeguarding. The Digital Legacy Association was founded by James Norris, who is one of the authors of this book (Norris, 2024). Since 2015, the Digital Legacy Association has led initiatives (such as training, campaigning, think tanks, providing resources and providing best practice frameworks) to support public and professionals with the skills and resources to support best practice in digital assets planning and digital legacy safeguarding (Fig. 10.4).

Fig. 10.4 The logo of the Digital Legacy Association. *Credit* The Digital Legacy Association

The Digital Legacy Association

The Digital Legacy Association coordinates an international Digital Death Survey (most recently completed in 2025) and uses this information to generate a Digital Death Report. The Not for Profit organisation and the data collected helps to inform guidance frameworks and strategies for international governmental and non-governmental organizations (Norris and Sofka, 2025). They provide expert teaching at international academic events, and the Digital Legacy Association coordinates an annual Digital Legacy Conference, where expert speakers provide thought leadership for multi-professional audiences. The Digital Legacy Association are also an observer for the European Law Institute's 'Model Rules on Succession of Digital Assets, Data and other Digital Remains' program (https://digitallegacyassociation.org/european-law-institute-digital-assets-project).

James is also the founder of MyWishes (https://www.mywishes.co.uk), which is a free to use, 'tech for good' platform. On the 'MyWishes' online platform, users are supported to write their Last Will & Testament, safeguard their digital legacy, plan for their funeral, curate a bucket list (a list of the things that a person would like to do or achieve before they die), leave goodbye messages and to complete an ACP (MyWishes, 2025).

As part of MyWishes public health campaigning, MyWishes launched the UK's first Advance Care Plan Day in 2024 to raise awareness about the importance of Advance Care Planning (https://advancecareplanday.org/). The event was successful, and the UK Advance Care Plan Day is now observed annually (Figs. 10.5 and 10.6).

Further information about all aspects of the work of the Digital Legacy Association, (including free resources, the Digital Death Reports and information about the Digital Legacy Conference) is freely available from the following websites:

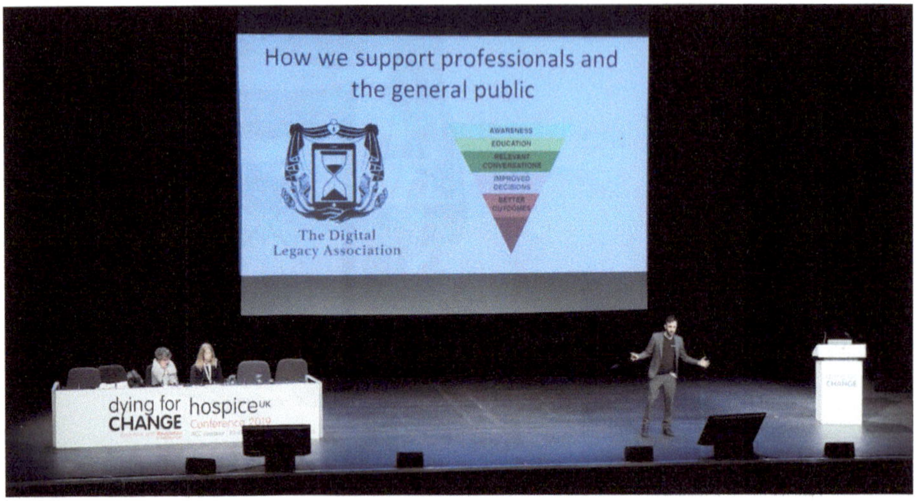

Fig. 10.5 James Norris (founder of the Digital Legacy Association) speaking at the Hospice UK conference. *Credit* The Digital Legacy Association

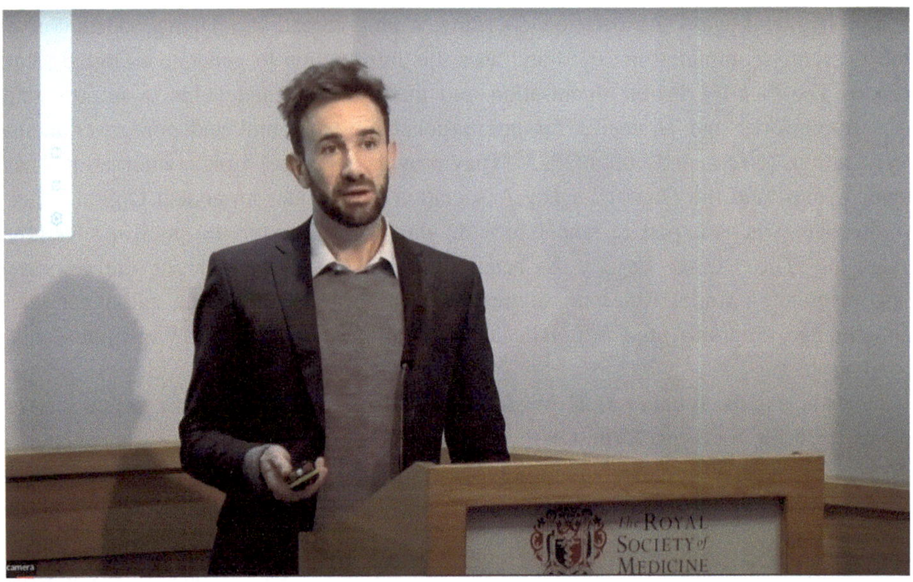

Fig. 10.6 James Norris (founder of the digital legacy association) speaking at the Royal Society of Medicine. *Credit* The Digital Legacy Association

https://digitallegacyassociation.org.
https://www.mywishes.co.uk.
https://advancecareplanday.org.

10.14 The Future of Funerals

Traditionally, the experience of losing a loved one is often accompanied by ritualistic and spiritual practices, which serve as a way for people to mourn the loss and begin the grieving process (MacNeil et al., 2023). Physical distancing limitations enforced by the COVID-19 pandemic caused grieving families and funeral providers to host funerals online (Pitsillides and Wallace, 2021). Although the pandemic has now ended, there is public recognition of positives and negative aspects of live-streamed funerals, with evidence that this practice will continue (Rawlings et al., 2024, Norris and Sofka, 2025). For example, data from the 2025 Digital Death Report indicates that only 10% of respondents objected to the idea of a close family member viewing a live-video stream of their funeral instead of attending in-person, which may suggest evolving societal attitudes towards funeral streaming (when compared to 2016 data where 54% respondents objected) (Norris and Sofka, 2025). Future developments in cultural practices in virtual funeral attendance will likely involve greater use of virtual reality (VR) and augmented reality (AR), as these technologies provide an immersive experience for people to develop new rituals to remember the dead and support the bereaved (Leng et al., 2023). Virtual memorials will likely become increasingly personalised with advances in other technologies, such as 3D printing (also known as an additive manufacturing device, which creates three-dimensional objects by layering materials, typically plastic, resin, or metal, according to a digital model (Gokhare et al., 2017)), which has been used to reconstruct faces of deceased people (where their faces have been damaged by trauma) so friends and family can view the body in the mortuary (South China Morning Post, 2021). 3D printing can potentially be used for other funeral practices, such as customizing urns, caskets, or memorial sculptures. Furthermore, other digital technologies will continue to be incorporated into different funeral rituals, as digital guestbooks, digital photos, video, holograms and pre-recorded (or AI generated) messages from the deceased (Norris and Sofka, 2025).

10.15 The Future of Grieving and the Digital Afterlife

Grief is a process which will affect everyone in a different way. There is a growing evidence to suggest that continuing bonds with a deceased person can provide comfort in the grieving process (Klass et al., 2014). Traditionally this may have been through looking at photographs or watching videos. With advancing technology there are opportunities to use AI to create digital replicas or avatars of the deceased based on their digital footprints (e.g., social media posts, emails, photos, and videos) (Norris and Sofka, 2025).

AI is increasingly being used to preserve the memory of the dead, by creating a digital representation of a deceased person (an avatar). AI allows a living person to interact with the 'avatar' of a dead person. For example, an AI computer program can be used to mimic the writing style of a dead person. Another example is the use of a computer to create a hologram of the deceased, to mimic their appearance, movements, and voice (Hollanek and Nowaczyk-Basińska, 2024). These avatars may mimic the person's speech patterns, personality traits, and mannerisms to create a convincing simulation of their presence. Digital avatars may be created with a view to providing emotional support and companionship to those who are grieving, offering a sense of connection with the deceased (Braman et al., 2011). It is possible for people (both the individual in question and those important) to proactively use technologies (such as AI, VR and LLM) to prepare their 'digital afterlife' to preserve human consciousness (or identity) in a digital form beyond physical death. This creates the potential for the 'essence' of the deceased person to live forever (digital immortality) in the digital world, meaning they can continue to develop interests, engage with others and communicate their 'legacy' to the living (Öhman and Floridi, 2017). Potential benefits of living people interacting with avatars of the deceased people include the possibility to interact with historical figures (e.g., Leonardo Da Vinci has been recreated as an AI chatbot (Pataranutaporn et al., 2023)), to engage with deceased friends and family, to receive a message at a specified time from the avatar of the deceased (e.g., a person may receive message from a deceased family member on their 18th birthday) (Morse, 2024). However, it is also possible that interactions with avatars of the deceased may be harmful for individuals, creating sociological and ethical questions about the 'essence' and ownership of a person. For example, who owns your face, your voice, your writing style or speech prosody after death? What makes the 'essence' of a person special, and unique, if these attributes can be recreated by a machine after death? What are the consequences of a 'second death' if the digital avatar is 'switched off' or deleted? (Savin-Baden and Mason-Robbie, 2020). Consequently, debates about the intricacies of AI avatars of the deceased are complex, and future work is needed to explore how AI grief tech should be used, to understand public opinion, and to determine the important sociological, legal and ethical issues associated with these technologies (Hollanek and Nowaczyk-Basińska, 2024; Norris and Sofka, 2025; Braman et al., 2011, Morse, 2024).

10.16 Climate Considerations for AgeTech in Palliative Care

It is important to consider the environmental impact which may result from AgeTech. The volume of electronic waste (e-waste) is growing globally, which is challenging as discarded electronic and electronic waste is hazardous and challenging to recycle (Perkins et al., 2014). The amount of healthcare e-waste is increasing and will likely further continue, due to the developments discussed in this book (Bandyopadhyay et al., 2022). Future work should identify sustainability requirements for AgeTech, and development of e-waste management initiatives specific to the healthcare sector, such as reusing, repurposing and recycling devices (Lefebvre et al., 2011; Bandyopadhyay et al., 2022). A particular challenge for palliative care AgeTech is how to use devices and systems, which have been designed to meet the specific needs of individuals, thus preventing their ability to be reused. Furthermore, there may be reluctance for some individuals to use AgeTech devices after the death of its previous user.

It is important to consider the potential climate related impact of increasing energy-use from cloud storage of data of the dead (Justin Adamson, 2017). It is possible that people will arrange for their data to remain accessible for others after death, which will require data to be stored in electronic cloud servers (e.g. Google Drive, OneDrive, Facebook, Instagram etc. etc.) (Mél, 2021). The expansion of societies' after-death existence, with increased energy-intensive cloud-storage of data, may contribute to global emissions which are warming the climate (Tennison et al., 2021). Consideration of how data should be archived or deleted may have ethical considerations; for example, who is responsible for archiving human history and what are the consequences of deleting data of the deceased? Therefore, future work is needed to further understand the energy, storage and climate implications of the digital afterlife and to consider opportunities to revolutionize energy management (e.g., through advancements in quantum computing and nuclear fusion) (Fontana, 2024).

10.17 Conclusions

The purpose of this book is not to provide a complete overview of the different types of AgeTech technologies available (as the development of these technologies have evolved as we wrote this book, and continue to evolve as you read these words); but to provide insight and discussion of the specific needs that people, with serious life-limiting illness have and how technologies could potentially be used to meet these needs.

In this book we have outlined several possible, person-focused, areas where technologies can potentially support the holistic care of older people with palliative care needs. Many of these innovations are exciting and provide the possibility of a future where AgeTech is used to maintain independence, provide support, personalize treatment, facilitate communication and widen access to healthcare. However, we have also identified challenges that need to be considered, such as the efficacy and effectiveness of AgeTech, prohibitive costs, inequality of access and risk of harm through inappropriate use. Consequently, it is important for the reader to carefully consider the current landscape, and determine the current opportunities and challenges of AgeTech in palliative care, to ensure that future work focuses on ensuring its meaningful use in improving care of older people with serious illness.

References

Abel, J. & Taubert, M. 2020. Coronavirus pandemic: compassionate communities and information technology. *BMJ Supportive & Palliative Care,* 10, 369–371.

Ahmad, K. A. B., Khujamatov, H., Akhmedov, N., Bajuri, M. Y., Ahmad, M. N. & Ahmadian, A. 2022. Emerging trends and evolutions for smart city healthcare systems. *Sustainable Cities and Society,* 80, 103695.

Allsop, M. J., Powell, R. A. & Namisango, E. 2018. The state of mHealth development and use by palliative care services in sub-Saharan Africa: a systematic review of the literature. *BMJ supportive & palliative care,* 8, 155–163.

Bajwa, J., Munir, U., Nori, A. & Williams, B. 2021. Artificial intelligence in healthcare: transforming the practice of medicine. *Future Healthcare Journal,* 8, e188–e194.

Baldassarre, D., Piazza, O. & Mcconnell, P. 2023. Emerging ethical challenges in healthcare in the 21st century. *Anaesthesia & Intensive Care Medicine,* 24, 729–732.

Bandyopadhyay, A., Chatterjee, R. & Das, N. 2022. E-Waste Management in Digital Healthcare System and Sustainability Paradigm. *Environmental Informatics: Challenges and Solutions.* Springer.

Beauchamp, T. L. & Childress, J. F. 1994. *Principles of biomedical ethics,* Edicoes Loyola.

Bettini, E. A. 2020. COVID-19 Pandemic Restrictions and the Use of Technology for Pediatric Palliative Care in the Acute Care Setting. *J Hosp Palliat Nurs,* 22, 432–434.

Bone, A. E., Gomes, B., Etkind, S. N., Verne, J., Murtagh, F. E. M., Evans, C. J. & Higginson, I., J. 2017. What is the impact of population ageing on the future provision of end-of-life care? Population-based projections of place of death. *Palliative Medicine,* 32, 329–336.

Braman, J., Dudley, A. & Vincenti, G. Death, social networks and virtual worlds: a look into the digital afterlife. 2011 ninth international conference on software engineering research, management and applications, 2011. IEEE, 186–192.

Calton, B., Abedini, N. & Fratkin, M. 2020. Telemedicine in the Time of Coronavirus. *J Pain Symptom Manage,* 60, e12–e14.

Carbonell, J. G., Michalski, R. S. & Mitchell, T. M. 1983. An overview of machine learning.

Chávarri-Guerra, Y., Ramos-López, W. A., Covarrubias-Gómez, A., Sánchez-Román, S., Quiroz-Friedman, P., Alcocer-Castillejos, N., del Pilar Milke-García, M., Carrillo-Soto, M., Morales-Alfaro, A. & Medina-Palma, M. 2020. Providing Supportive and Palliative Care Using Telemedicine for Patients with Advanced Cancer During the COVID-19 Pandemic in Mexico. *The oncologist.*

Chen, C., Garrido, T., Chock, D., Okawa, G. & Liang, L. 2009. The Kaiser Permanente Electronic Health Record: transforming and streamlining modalities of care. *Health Aff (Millwood),* 28, 323–33.

Chonko, L. 2012. Ethical theories. *Retrieved [14th October, 2020] from* https://www.dsrf.org/wp-content/uploads/2012/07/EthicalTheories.pdf.

Chua, I. S., Jackson, V. & Kamdar, M. 2020. Webside Manner during the COVID-19 Pandemic: Maintaining Human Connection during Virtual Visits. *J Palliat Med,* 23, 1507–1509.

Collins, B. 2016. Big Data and Health Economics: Strengths, Weaknesses, Opportunities and Threats. *PharmacoEconomics,* 34, 101–106.

Cook, D. J., Duncan, G., Sprint, G. & Fritz, R. L. 2018. Using smart city technology to make healthcare smarter. *Proceedings of the IEEE,* 106, 708–722.

Coughlan, D. 2021. Physical activity and the insurance industry. BMJ Publishing Group Ltd.

Crosby, B., Hanchanale, S., Stanley, S. & Nwosu, A. C. 2021. Evaluating the use of video communication technology in a hospital specialist palliative care team during the COVID-19 pandemic. *AMRC Open Research,* 3, 5.

Department of Health Social Care 2018. The future of healthcare: our vision for digital, data and technology in health and care. https://www.gov.uk/government/publications/the-future-of-healthcare-our-vision-for-digital-data-and-technology-in-health-and-care/the-future-of-healthcare-our-vision-for-digital-data-and-technology-in-health-and-care: DHSC London.

Esteva, A., Kuprel, B., Novoa, R. A., Ko, J., Swetter, S. M., Blau, H. M. & Thrun, S. 2017. Dermatologist-level classification of skin cancer with deep neural networks. *Nature,* 542, 115–118.

Etkind, S. N., Bone, A. E., Gomes, B., Lovell, N., Evans, C. J., HIGGINSON, I. J. & MURTAGH, F. E. M. 2017. How many people will need palliative care in 2040? Past trends, future projections and implications for services. *BMC Medicine,* 15, 102.

Finucane, A., O'Donnell, H., Lugton, J., Swenson, C. & Pagliari, C. 2020. Digital Health Interventions in Palliative Care: A Systematic Meta-Review and Evidence Synthesis. *medRxiv,* 2020.09.16.20195834.

Flores, S., Abrukin, L., Jiang, L., Titone, L., Firew, T., Lee, J., Gavin, N., Romney, M.-L., Nakagawa, S. & Chang, B. P. 2020. Novel Use of Telepalliative Care in a New York City Emergency Department During the COVID-19 Pandemic. *The Journal of emergency medicine,* 59, 714–716.

Floridi, L. 2023. The ethics of artificial intelligence: Principles, challenges, and opportunities.

Fontana, C. 2024. Energy Management Systems and Potential Applications of Quantum Computing in the Energy Sector.

Gillon, R. 1994. Medical ethics: four principles plus attention to scope. *Bmj,* 309, 184.

Gillon, R. 2015. Defending the four principles approach as a good basis for good medical practice and therefore for good medical ethics. *Journal of medical ethics,* 41, 111–116.

Gokhare, V. G., Raut, D. & Shinde, D. 2017. A review paper on 3D-printing aspects and various processes used in the 3D-printing. *Int. J. Eng. Res. Technol,* 6, 953–958.

Gomes, N., Pato, M., Lourenço, A. R. & Datia, N. 2023. A survey on wearable sensors for mental health monitoring. *Sensors,* 23, 1330.

Greene, C. S., Tan, J., Ung, M., Moore, J. H. & Cheng, C. 2014. Big data bioinformatics. *J Cell Physiol,* 229, 1896–900.

Grewal, U. S., Terauchi, S. & Beg, M. S. 2020. Telehealth and Palliative Care for Patients With Cancer: Implications of the COVID-19 Pandemic. *JMIR Cancer,* 6, e20288.

Haghi, M., Thurow, K. & Stoll, R. 2017. Wearable Devices in Medical Internet of Things: Scientific Research and Commercially Available Devices. *Healthc Inform Res,* 23, 4–15.

Harris, D. A., Archbald-Pannone, L., Kaur, J., Cattell-Gordon, D., Rheuban, K. S., Ombres, R. L., Albero, K., Steele, R., Bell, T. D. & Mutter, J. B. 2021. Rapid Telehealth-Centered Response to COVID-19 Outbreaks in Postacute and Long-Term Care Facilities. *Telemedicine and e-Health,* 27, 102–106.

Hollanek, T. & Nowaczyk-Basińska, K. 2024. Griefbots, Deadbots, Postmortem Avatars: on Responsible Applications of Generative AI in the Digital Afterlife Industry. *Philosophy & Technology,* 37, 1–22.

Jung, Y. 2017. Hybrid-aware model for senior wellness service in smart home. *Sensors,* 17, 1182.

Justin Adamson. 2017. *Carbon and the Cloud* [Online]. Medium. Available: https://medium.com/stanford-magazine/carbon-and-the-cloud-d6f481b79dfe [Accessed 6th June 2024].

Kasket, E. 2019. *All the ghosts in the machine: The digital afterlife of your personal data,* Hachette UK.

Klass, D., Silverman, P. R. & Nickman, S. 2014. *Continuing bonds: New understandings of grief,* Taylor & Francis.

Lal, A., Bell, G., Curseen, K. & Kavalieratos, D. 2020. Teaching Telepalliative Care: An Elective Rotation for Medical Students during the COVID-19 Pandemic. *Journal of Palliative Medicine.*

Lally, K., Kematick, B. S., Gorman, D. & Tulsky, J. 2021. Rapid Conversion of a Palliative Care Outpatient Clinic to Telehealth. *JCO Oncol Pract,* 17, e62–e67.

Lefebvre, E., Romero, A. & Lefebvre, L.-A. 2011. E-Waste In The Healthcare Sector: A Growing International Problem. *International Journal of Arts & Sciences,* 4, 21.

Leng, P., Lang, X. & Pan, Z. The Future Value of the Metaverse for Funeral and Interment. 2023 International Conference on the Cognitive Computing and Complex Data (ICCD), 2023. IEEE, 334–339.

Liu, L., Stroulia, E., Nikolaidis, I., Miguel-Cruz, A. & Rios Rincon, A. 2016. Smart homes and home health monitoring technologies for older adults: A systematic review. *Int J Med Inform,* 91, 44–59.

Lu, Y., Xie, D., Zhang, X., Dong, S., Zhang, H., Yu, B., Wang, G., Wang, J. J. & Li, L. 2020. Management of intractable pain in patients with implanted spinal cord stimulation devices during the COVID-19 pandemic using a remote and wireless programming system. *Frontiers in neuroscience,* 14.

Mackey, R. M., Yeow, M. E., Christensen, A. R., Ingram, C., Carey, E. C. & Lapid, M. I. 2020. Reconnecting: Strategies for Supporting Isolated Older Adults during COVID-19 through Telepalliative Care. *Clinical gerontologist,* 1–8.

Macneil, A., Findlay, B., Bimman, R., Hocking, T., Barclay, T. & Ho, J. 2023. Exploring the use of virtual funerals during the COVID-19 pandemic: A scoping review. *OMEGA-Journal of Death and Dying,* 88, 425–448.

Mél Hogan. 2021. *The Future of Death (in the Cloud)* [Online]. Website of Network in Canadian History & Environment (NiCHE). Available: https://niche-canada.org/2021/03/08/the-future-of-death-in-the-cloud/ [Accessed 6th June 2024].

Mills, J., Li, C., Fullerton, S., Chapman, M., Jap, J., Sinclair, C., Collins, A. & Campbell, E. 2020. Staying connected and informed: Online resources and virtual communities of practice supporting palliative care during the novel coronavirus pandemic. *Progress in Palliative Care,* 28, 251–253.

Mills, J., Fox, J., Damarell, R., Tieman, J. & Yates, P. 2021a. Palliative care providers' use of digital health and perspectives on technological innovation: a national study. *BMC Palliat Care,* 20, 124.

Mills, J., Kim, S.-H., Chan, H. Y., Ho, M.-H., Montayre, J., Liu, M. F. & Lin, C.-C. 2021b. Palliative care education in the Asia Pacific: Challenges and progress towards palliative care development. Taylor & Francis.

Morse, T. 2024. Digital necromancy: Users' perceptions of digital afterlife and posthumous communication technologies. *Information, Communication & Society,* 27, 240–256.

MyWishes. 2025. *Website of MyWishes* [Online]. Available: https://www.mywishes.co.uk/ [Accessed 27th March 2025].

Ngoma, M., Mushi, B., Morse, R. S., Ngoma, T., Mahuna, H., Lambden, K., Quinn, E., Sagan, S. B., Ho, Y. X. & Lucas, F. L. 2021. mPalliative Care Link: Examination of a Mobile Solution to Palliative Care Coordination Among Tanzanian Patients With Cancer. *JCO Global Oncology,* 7, 1306–1315.

Niki, K., Okamoto, Y. & Ueda, M. 2020. Response to Wang et al., Virtual Reality as a Bridge in Palliative Care during COVID-19 (https://doi.org/10.1089/jpm.2020.0212). *J Palliat Med,* 23**,** 892–894.

Nkhoma, K. B., Ebenso, B., Akeju, D., Adejoh, S., Bennett, M., Chirenje, M., Dandadzi, A., Nabirye, E., Namukwaya, E. & Namisango, E. 2021. Stakeholder perspectives and requirements to guide the development of digital technology for palliative cancer services: a multi-country, cross-sectional, qualitative study in Nigeria, Uganda and Zimbabwe. *BMC palliative care,* 20**,** 1–16.

Norris, J. & Sofka, C. 2025. *Digital Death Report 2025—Digital Legacy Association* [Online]. Available: https://digitallegacyassociation.org/about/reports-2/ [Accessed].

Norris, J. 2020. *Tablets Against Loneliness* [Online]. Available: https://tabletsagainstloneliness.co.uk [Accessed 24th March 2025].

Norris, J. 2024. *Website of James Norris* [Online]. Available: https://www.jamesnorris.me/ [Accessed 1st June 2024].

Nowaczyk-Basińska, K. 2025. Digital afterlife leaders: professionalisation as a social innovation in the digital afterlife industry. *Mortality***,** 1–22.

Nwosu, A. C., Collins, B. & Mason, S. 2018. Big Data analysis to improve care for people living with serious illness: The potential to use new emerging technology in palliative care. *Palliative Medicine,* 32**,** 164–166.

Nwosu, A. C., Mcglinchey, T., Sanders, J., Stanley, S., Palfrey, J., Lubbers, P., Chapman, L., Finucane, A. & Mason, S. 2022. Identification of digital health priorities for palliative care research: modified delphi study. *JMIR aging,* 5**,** e32075.

Nwosu, A. C. 2023. Telehealth requires improved evidence to achieve its full potential in palliative care. SAGE Publications Sage UK: London, England.

Öhman, C. & Floridi, L. 2017. The political economy of death in the age of information: A critical approach to the digital afterlife industry. *Minds and machines,* 27**,** 639–662.

Pataranutaporn, P., Danry, V., Blanchard, L., Thakral, L., Ohsugi, N., Maes, P. & Sra, M. Living memories: AI-generated characters as digital mementos. Proceedings of the 28th International Conference on Intelligent User Interfaces, 2023. 889–901.

Perkins, D. N., Drisse, M.-N. B., Nxele, T. & Sly, P. D. 2014. E-waste: a global hazard. *Annals of global health,* 80**,** 286–295.

PITSILLIDES, S. & WALLACE, J. 2021. Physically distant but socially connected: Streaming funerals, memorials and ritual design during COVID-19. *Death, grief and loss in the context of COVID-19***,** 60–76.

Rawlings, D., Miller-Lewis, L. & Tieman, J. 2024. Impact of the COVID-19 pandemic on funerals: Experiences of participants in the 2020 Dying2Learn massive open online course. *OMEGA-journal of Death and Dying,* 89**,** 429–451.

Ritchey, K. C., Foy, A., Mcardel, E. & Gruenewald, D. A. 2020. Reinventing palliative care delivery in the era of covid-19: how telemedicine can support end of life care. *American Journal of Hospice and Palliative Medicine®,* 37**,** 992–997.

Samara, J., Liu, W.-M., Kroon, W., Harvie, B., Hingeley, R. & Johnston, N. 2021. Telehealth Palliative Care Needs Rounds During a Pandemic. *The Journal for Nurse Practitioners.*

Sansom-Daly, U. M. & Bradford, N. 2020. Grappling with the 'human' problem hiding behind the technology: Telehealth during and beyond COVID-19. *Psycho-oncology.*

Savin-Baden, M. & Mason-Robbie, V. 2020. *Digital afterlife: Death matters in a digital age,* CRC Press.

Sleeman, K. E., de Brito, M., Etkind, S., Nkhoma, K., Guo, P., Higginson, I. J., Gomes, B. & Harding, R. 2019. The escalating global burden of serious health-related suffering: projections to 2060 by world regions, age groups, and health conditions. *The Lancet Global Health,* 7**,** e883–e892.

Sofka, C. 2012. *Dying, death, and grief in an online universe: For counselors and educators*, Springer Publishing Company.

South China Morning Post. 2021. *China's funeral parlours use 3D printing to restore faces of the dead destroyed by tragedy, revolutionise mortuary practice* [Online]. Website of the South China Morning Post. Available: https://www.scmp.com/news/people-culture/social-welfare/article/3129498/chinas-funeral-parlours-use-3d-printing-restore [Accessed 22nd March 2025].

Stanley, S., Finucane, A., Thompson, A. & Nwosu, A. C. 2024. How can technology be used to support communication in palliative care beyond the covid-19 pandemic: a mixed-methods national survey of palliative care healthcare professionals. *BMC palliative care,* 23**,** 40.

Taylor, R., Norris, J., Mckay, P., West, C. & Wade, K. 2021. 'the room where it happens': An exploration of personalised virtual reality (VR)-bringing the home to the hospice during the covid-19 pandemic. *Palliative Medicine***,** 120–120.

Tennison, I., Roschnik, S., Ashby, B., Boyd, R., Hamilton, I., Oreszczyn, T., Owen, A., Romanello, M., Ruyssevelt, P. & Sherman, J. D. 2021. Health care's response to climate change: a carbon footprint assessment of the NHS in England. *The Lancet Planetary Health,* 5**,** e84–e92.

The Digital Legacy Association. 2024. *The Digital Legacy Association* [Online]. The website of the Digital Legacy Association. Available: https://digitallegacyassociation.org/ [Accessed 2025].

The Health Foundation. 2014. *Insight 2014: Informatics to identify and inform best practice in out of hours secondary care* [Online]. The website of the Health Foundation. Available: http://www.health.org.uk/programmes/projects/insight-2014-informatics-identify-and-inform-best-practice-out-hours-secondary [Accessed].

Topol, E. 2019. Preparing the Healthcare Workforce to Deliver the Digital Future the Topol Review: An Independent Report on Behalf of the Secretary of State for Health and Social Care. *NHS Health Education: London, UK.*

Varkey, B. 2021. Principles of clinical ethics and their application to practice. *Medical Principles and Practice,* 30**,** 17–28.

Wang, S. S., Teo, W. Z., Teo, W. Z. & Chai, Y. W. 2020. Virtual reality as a bridge in palliative care during COVID-19. *Journal of palliative medicine,* 23**,** 756–756.

Wherton, J., Shaw, S., Papoutsi, C., Seuren, L. & Greenhalgh, T. 2020. Guidance on the introduction and use of video consultations during COVID-19: important lessons from qualitative research. *BMJ Leader***,** leader-2020-000262.

Wise, J. 2023. Covid-19: WHO declares end of global health emergency. British Medical Journal Publishing Group.

Yu, K.-H., Zhang, C., Berry, G. J., Altman, R. B., Ré, C., Rubin, D. L. & Snyder, M. 2016. Predicting non-small cell lung cancer prognosis by fully automated microscopic pathology image features. 7**,** 12474.

MIX
Papier aus verantwortungsvollen Quellen
Paper from responsible sources
FSC® C105338

If you have any concerns about our products,
you can contact us on
ProductSafety@springernature.com

In case Publisher is established outside the EU,
the EU authorized representative is:
Springer Nature Customer Service Center GmbH
Europaplatz 3, 69115 Heidelberg, Germany

Printed by Libri Plureos GmbH
in Hamburg, Germany